Diana Murphy

OPTAVIA
DIET COOKBOOK

200+ Healthy, Easy, And Super Energetic Recipes to

Burn Fat and Lose Weight Fast. The Complete Guide to

A Long-Term Trasformation With Lean and Green Meals

© Copyright 2020 - All rights reserved.

Table of Contents

Introduction

The Optavia Diet is the brainchild of one Rohan Patel, who in the year 2008, had suffered from a heart attack. Patel was advised to consume foods that were low in fat and cholesterol. Though he did try to adopt a low-fat diet, it was a challenge for him. He was a businessman, and had a very hectic schedule and was unable to maintain a strict diet for long. Rohan Patel succeeded in losing weight, but found that he had a difficult time with eating and decided to present this as an alternative. Throughout the years 2008 and 2009, the Optavia Diet was planned and conceptualized.

The actual diet product was given a name – Optavia. The popular phrase that he used was "Having Optavia is better than having no diet!" Patel worked upon the smaller plan of the diet – '5 & 1' that has been proved very effective by various researchers and dieticians. The five parts of the '5 & 1' program are small meals and consists of five portions of a specific food, while the sixth part of the program involves the consumption of carbohydrates for energy. It's a good idea to have the right amount of carbohydrates, which can spark weight loss.

The Optavia diet was soon ready to be launched in 2010. While the product is easy to consume, it is not to be mistaken as a weight-loss food. The product is not meant to be consumed by anyone and everyone who wishes to lose weight. It's a strict diet program that is meant for individuals who know the importance of health and the body and who are looking for a better way to lose weight. The product is only meant for consuming a single meal a day and not several small ones at a time. It is a popular way of consuming your food for those who are short on time. Though it has been termed an "easy start" approach to losing weight, it is not easy to achieve. Following '5 & 1' each day and using energy enhancers is not easy. Optavia insists that dieticians and consultants are employed by every individual who desires to try the diet out.

The Optavia Diet is not meant for a specific community but aims to cater to individuals who choose to avoid "overanalyzing" an eating schedule. Five out of the six small meals a day are pre-planned and pre-packaged with Optavia's famous '5 & 1' plan, removing the need for any major choices when it's time to feed. Optavia happens to be a choice of individuals with a packed schedule, but the reduced-calorie strategy of the product is meant for anybody who wishes to lose weight. As a diet product, a strict lifestyle is expected on the part of the consumer who wishes to follow the diet.

Priced at $70 for the selected starter kit, Optavia claims that they are the only one in the market offering a package including weight loss consultants and dieticians.

CHAPTER 1:

What is the Optavia Diet

The Optavia diet is a practice that aims to reduce or maintain current weight. It is a diet that recommends eating a combination of processed foods called fuellings and home-cooked meals (lean and green meals). It is believed that it sticks to the brand product (input) and supplements it with meat, vegetables, and fatty snacks; this will keep you satisfied and nourished. At the same time you don't need to worry much about losing muscles because you are eating enough protein and consuming too few calories. And that way, the individual who practices the diet can lose around 12 pounds in just 12 weeks using the ideal 5&1 weight plan.

In short, the Optavian diet is a program that focuses on cutting calories and reducing carbohydrates in meals. To do this effectively, combine packaged foods called fuels with home-cooked meals, which encourages weight loss.

The Optavia Diet encourages people to limit the number of calories that they should take daily. Under this program, dieters are encouraged to consume between 800 and 1000 calories daily. But unlike other types of commercial diet regimens, the Optavia Diet comes in different variations. There are currently three variations of the Optavia Diet plan that one can choose from according to one's needs.

Different Optavia Diet program

- **5&1 Optavia Diet Plan:** This is the most common version of the Optavia Diet, and it involves eating five prepackaged meals from the Optimal Health Fuelings and one home-made balanced meal.

- **4&2&1 Octavia Diet Plan:** This diet plan is designed for people who want to have flexibility while following this regimen. Under this program, dieters are encouraged to eat more calories and have more flexible food choices. This means that they can consume 4 prepackaged Optimal Health Fuelings food, three home-cooked meals from the Lean and Green, and one snack daily.

- **5&2&2 Optavia Diet Plan:** This diet plan is perfect for individuals who prefer to have a flexible meal plan in order to achieve a healthy weight. It is recommended for a wide variety of people. Under this diet regimen, dieters are required to eat 5 fuelings, 2 lean and green meals, and 2 healthy snacks.

- **3&3 Optavia Diet Plan:** This particular Diet plan is created for people who have moderate weight problems and merely want to maintain a healthy body. Under this diet plan, dieters are encouraged to consume 3 prepackaged Optimal Health Fuelings and three home-cooked meals.

- **Optavia for Nursing Mothers:** This diet regimen is designed for nursing mothers with babies of at least two months old. Aside from supporting breastfeeding mothers, it also encourages gradual weight loss.

- **Optavia for Diabetes:** This Optavia Diet plan is designed for people who have Type 1 and Type 2 diabetes. The meal plans are designed so that dieters consume more green and lean meals, depending on their needs and condition.

- **Optavia for Gout:** This diet regimen incorporates a balance of foods that are low in purines and moderate in protein.

- **Optavia for Seniors (65 years and older):** Designed for seniors, this Optavia Diet plan has some variations following the components of Fuelings depending on the needs and activities of the senior dieters.

- **Optavia for Teen Boys and Optavia for Teen Girls (13-18 years old):** Designed for active teens, the Optavia for Teens Boys and Optavia for Teens Girls provide the right nutrition to growing teens.

Regardless of which type of Optavia Diet plan you choose, it is important that you talk with a coach to help you determine which plan is right for you based on your individual goals.

- **How to Start This Diet**

The Optavia Diet is comprised of different phases. A certified coach will educate you on the steps that you need to undertake if you want to follow this regimen. Below are some of the things you need to know, especially when you are still starting with this diet regimen.

Initial Steps

During this phase, people are encouraged to consume 800 to 1,000 calories to help them shed off at least 12 pounds within the next 12 weeks. For instance, if you are following the 5&1 Optavia Diet Plan, then you need to eat 1 meal every 2 or 3 hours and include a 30-minute moderate workout most days of your week. You need to consume not more than 100 grams of Carbs daily during this phase.

Further, consuming meals are highly encouraged. This phase also encourages the dieter to include 1 optional snack per day, such as ½ cup sugar-free gelatin, 3 celery sticks, and 12 ounces nuts. Aside from these things, below are other things that you need to remember when following this phase:

- Make sure that the portion size recommendations are for cooked weight and not the raw weight of your ingredients

- Opt for meals that are baked, grilled, broiled, or poached. Avoid frying foods, as this will increase your calorie intake.

- Eat at least 2 servings of fish rich in Omega-3 fatty acids. These include fishes like tuna, salmon, trout, mackerel, herring, and other cold-water fishes.

- Choose meatless alternatives like tofu and tempeh.

- Follow the program even when you are dining out. Keep in mind that drinking alcohol is discouraged when following this plan.

Maintenance Phase

As soon as you have attained your desired weight, the next phase is the transition stage. It is a 6-week stage that involves increasing your calorie intake to 1,550 per day. This is also the phase when you are allowed to add more varieties into your meal, such as whole grains, low-fat dairy, and fruits.

After six weeks, you can now move into the 3&3 Optavia Diet plan, so you are required to eat three Lean and Green meals and 3 Fueling foods.

CHAPTER 2:

The Benefits of the Optavia Diet

Ideal for Portion Controllers - One of the hardest parts of the diet is learning to control portions and stick to them.

Practice long-term relationship with food: Guiding the community to follow the Optavia diet can help improve a long-term positive relationship with food. Over time, you come to realize the types of foods you are allowed to eat and appreciate the healthy options you have.

No Responsibility Partner Needed: While some diets encourage you to make a friend to the diet, the Optavia diet is ideal for people who have no responsibility partners. The point is that people are connected to a community of dietitians who can provide the necessary support during the phases of this diet.

Better Overall Health - This particular diet is known to help improve overall well-being. In addition to weight loss, several studies have also shown that the Optavia diet can help people maintain blood sugar levels and stable blood pressure due to the limited sodium intake in food. In fact, Optavia provides less than 2,300 milligrams of sodium a day.

A Deeper Look into the Optavia Diet

5&1 Optavia Diet Plan: This is the most common version of the Optavia Diet and it involves eating five prepackaged meals from the Optimal Health Fuelings and one home-made balanced meal.

4&2&1 Octavia Diet Plan: This diet plan is designed for people who want to have flexibility while following this regimen. Under this program, dieters are encouraged to eat more calories and have more flexible food choices. This means that they can consume 4 prepackaged Optimal Health Fuelings food, three home-cooked meals from the Lean and Green, and one snack daily.

5&2&2 Optavia Diet Plan: This diet plan is perfect for individuals who prefer to have a flexible meal plan in order to achieve a healthy weight. It is recommended for a wide variety of people. Under this diet regimen, dieters are required to eat 5 fuelings, 2 lean and green meals, and 2 healthy snacks.

3&3 Optavia Diet Plan: This particular Diet plan is created for people who have moderate weight problems and merely want to maintain a healthy body. Under this diet plan, dieters are encouraged to consume 3 prepackaged Optimal Health Fuelings and three home-cooked meals.

Optavia for Nursing Mothers: This diet regimen is designed for nursing mothers with babies of at least two months old. Aside from supporting breastfeeding mothers, it also encourages gradual weight loss.

Optavia for Diabetes: This Optavia Diet plan is designed for people who have Type 1 and Type 2 diabetes. The meal plans are designed so that dieters consume more green and lean meals depending on their needs and condition.

Optavia for Gout: This diet regimen incorporates a balance of foods that are low in purines and moderate in protein.

Optavia for old people (65 years and older): Designed for seniors, this Optavia Diet plan has some variations following the components of Fuelings depending on the needs and activities of the senior dieters.

Optavia for Teen Boys and Optavia for Teen Girls (13-18 years old): Designed for active teens, the Optavia for Teens Boys and Optavia for Teens Girls provide the right nutrition to growing teens.

CHAPTER 3:

How It Works

The Optavia diet is viewed as a high-protein diet, with its protein having 10–35% of your daily calories. Be that as it may, the handled, powdered kind can prompt some not exactly beautiful outcomes. "The protein confine in addition to added substances can cause you to feel enlarged and have caused some undesirable GI symptoms, making you off with unsweetened Greek yogurt for protein in a single smoothie," London says.

The FDA also doesn't direct dietary enhancements like shakes and powders for security and viability in a similar way it accomplishes for food. "Powders and protein 'mixes' may have unwanted fixings, or could interface with a drug you might be taking," London includes, "making it extra critical to ensure your doctor knows about you attempting the arrangement."

Like many commercial plans, Optavia involves buying most of the foods permitted on a diet in packaged form. The company deals on a wide range of food products that they call "fuelings"—on its website. These include pancakes, shakes, pasta dishes, soups, cookies, mashed potatoes, and popcorn.

Users pick the plan that best suits them. The 5 & 1 Plan entails eating five small meals per day. The meals can be selected from more than 60 substitutable fuelings, including one "lean and green" meal, probably veggies or protein that you will prepare by yourself. The Optimal Essential Kit, costing $356.15, provides 119 servings, or about 20 days' worth.

Is Optavia And Medifast The Same?

Relatively, Medifast Inc. is known as the parent company of Optavia. It also the owner and the one that operates the Medifast program. The program is already present in the '80s and '90s with doctors who prescribe meals to their clients. Optavia makes use of identical foods with a similar macronutrient profile. Consumers can sign up online for the plan by themselves.

How Much Does Optavia Cost?

In comparison, the United States Department of Agriculture estimates that a woman whose ages range from 10-50 can follow a nutritious diet while spending as little as $166.40 per month on groceries. As long as she is preparing all her meals at home.

How Nutritious Is Optavia Diet

Below is the breakdown comparison of meals' nutritional content on the Optavial Weight 5&1 Plan and the federal government's 2015 Dietary Guidelines for Americans.

	Optimal Weight 5&1 Plan	Federal Government Recommendation
Calories	800-1,000	Men 19-25: 2,800 26-45: 2,600 46-65: 2,400 65+: 2,200 Women 19-25: 2,200 26-50: 2,000 51+: 1,800
Total fat % of Calorie Intake	20%	20%-35%
Total Carbohydrates % of Calorie Intake	40%	45%-65%
Sugars	10%-20%	N/A
Fiber	25 g – 30 g	Men 19-30: 34 g. 31-50: 31 g. 51+: 28 g. Women 19-30: 28 g. 31-50: 25 g. 51+: 22 g.
Protein	40%	10%-35%
Sodium	Under 2,300 mg	Under 2,300 mg.
Potassium	Average 3,000 mg	At least 4,700 mg.
Calcium	1,000 mg – 1,200 mg	Men 1,000 mg. Women 19-50: 1,000 mg. 51+: 1,200 mg.

CHAPTER 4:

What can I Eat

There are many foods that you can eat while following the Optavia Diet. However, you must know these foods by heart. This is particularly true if you are just new to this diet, and you have to strictly follow the 5&1 Optavia Diet Plan.

Thus, this section is dedicated to the types of foods that are recommended and those to avoid while following this diet regimen.

Recommended foods

There are numerous categories of foods that can be eaten under this diet regimen. This section will break down the Lean and Green foods that you can eat while following this diet regime.

Lean Foods

Leanest Foods - These foods are considered to be the leanest as it has only up to 4 grams of total fat. Moreover, dieters should eat a 7-ounce cooked portion of these foods. Consume these foods with 1 healthy fat serving.

- **Fish:** Flounder, cod, haddock, grouper, Mahi, tilapia, tuna (yellowfin fresh or canned), and wild catfish.
- **Shellfish:** Scallops, lobster, crabs, shrimp
- **Game meat:** Elk, deer, buffalo
- **Ground turkey or other meat:** Should be 98% lean
- **Meatless alternatives:**14 egg whites, 2 cups egg substitute, 5 ounces seitan, 1 ½ cups 1% cottage cheese, and 12 ounces non-fat 0% Greek yogurt

Leaner Foods - These foods contain 5 to 9 grams of total fat. Consume these foods with 1 healthy fat serving. Make sure to consume only 6 ounces of a cooked portion of these foods daily:

- **Fish:** Halibut, trout, and swordfish
- **Chicken:** White meat such as breasts as long as the skin is removed
- **Turkey:** Ground turkey as long as it is 95% to 97% lean.
- **Meatless options:**2 whole eggs plus 4 egg whites, 2 whole eggs plus one cup egg substitute, 1 ½ cups 2% cottage cheese, and 12 ounces low fat 2% plain Greek yogurt

Lean Foods - These are foods that contain 10g to 20g total fat. When consuming these foods, there should be no serving of healthy fat. These include the following:

- **Fish:** Tuna (Bluefin steak), salmon, herring, farmed catfish, and mackerel
- **Lean beef:** Ground, steak, and roast
- **Lamb:** All cuts
- **Pork:** Pork chops, pork tenderloin, and all parts. Make sure to remove the skin
- **Ground turkey and other meats:**85% to 94% lean

- **Chicken:** Any dark meat
- **Meatless options:** 15 ounces extra-firm tofu, 3 whole eggs (up to two times per week), 4 ounces reduced-fat skim cheese, 8 ounces part-skim ricotta cheese, and 5 ounces tempeh

Healthy Fat Servings - Healthy fat servings are allowed under this diet. They should contain 5 grams of fat and less than grams of carbohydrates. Regardless of what type of Optavia Diet plan you follow, make sure that you add between 0 and 2 healthy fat servings daily. Below are the different healthy fat servings that you can eat:

- 1 teaspoon oil (any kind of oil)
- 1 tablespoon low carbohydrate salad dressing
- 2 tablespoons reduced-fat salad dressing
- 5 to 10 black or green olives
- 1 ½ ounce avocado
- 1/3-ounce plain nuts including peanuts, almonds, pistachios
- 1 tablespoon plain seeds such as chia, sesame, flax, and pumpkin seeds
- ½ tablespoon regular butter, mayonnaise, and margarine

Green Foods

This section will discuss the green servings that you still need to consume while following the Optavia Diet Plan. These include all kinds of vegetables that have been categorized from lower, moderate, and high in terms of carbohydrate content. One serving of vegetables should be at ½ cup unless otherwise specified.

Lower Carbohydrate - These are vegetables that contain low amounts of carbohydrates. If you are following the 5&1 Optavia Diet plan, then these vegetables are good for you.

- A cup of green leafy vegetables, such as collard greens (raw), lettuce (green leaf, iceberg, butterhead, and romaine), spinach (raw), mustard greens, spring mix, bok choy (raw), and watercress.
- ½ cup of vegetables including cucumbers, celery, radishes, white mushroom, sprouts (mung bean, alfalfa), arugula, turnip greens, escarole, nopales, Swiss chard (raw), jalapeno, and bok choy (cooked).

Moderate Carbohydrate - These are vegetables that contain moderate amounts of carbohydrates. Below are the types of vegetables that can be consumed in moderation:

- **½ cup of any of the following vegetables** such as asparagus, cauliflower, fennel bulb, eggplant, portabella mushrooms, kale, cooked spinach, summer squash (zucchini and scallop).

Higher Carbohydrates - Foods that are under this category contain a high amount of starch. Make sure to consume limited amounts of these vegetables.

- **½ cup of the following vegetables** like chayote squash, red cabbage, broccoli, cooked collard and mustard greens, green or wax beans, kohlrabi, kabocha squash, cooked leeks, any peppers, okra, raw scallion, summer squash such as straight neck and crookneck, tomatoes, spaghetti squash, turnips, jicama, cooked Swiss chard, and hearts of palm.

Foods to avoid

The following foods are to be avoided, except it's included in the fuelings — they include:

•Fried foods: meats, fish, shellfish, vegetables, desserts like baked goods

•Refined grains: white bread, pasta, scones, hotcakes, flour tortillas, wafers, white rice, treats, cakes, cakes

•Certain fats: margarine, coconut oil, strong shortening

•Whole fat dairy: milk, cheddar, yogurt

•Alcohol: all varieties, no exception

•Sugar-sweetened beverages: pop, natural product juice, sports drinks, caffeinated drinks, sweet tea

The accompanying nourishments are beyond reach while on the 5&1 plan, however, included back during the 6-week progress stage and permitted during the 3&3 plan:

•Fruit: all kinds of fresh fruits

•Low fat or without fat dairy: yogurt, milk, cheddar

CHAPTER 5:

What are the Fueling, and how do They Work in your Body

The food items from Optavia are Optavia Fuelings. Classic Fuelings, Essential Fuelings, and Select Fuelings are available. All and all, you may pick from over 60 products that provide calories in your journey to reducing weight.

Optavia Fuelings includes 24 high-quality, full proteins, lactic acid bacteria minerals and vitamins, and no artificial colors, flavors, or sweeteners. Optavia Select Fuelings has global-inspired recipes. The brand also employs non-GMO ingredients obtained from all over the world. You will select from 13 bold varieties and foreign flavors such as Bolivian chia seeds, Mediterranean rosemary, and Indonesian cinnamon. Your calorie restriction program would dictate the number of Fuelings that you consume per day.

- Fuel is a ready-made product, so you don't have to make anything at mealtime.
- You will participate and save cash on the goods as a coach and market them to anyone if you like.
- Having 60 or so fuels to pick from implies that you might eventually get tired of having the same food again and again.
- Must buy from a distributor of the company.

They claim items and services have been suggested and adopted by more than one million people for more than 20,000 clinicians. Nutritious, sweet, and efficient are Optavia Fuelings. At every point of the journey, they are clinically developed to have the best foods and are nutrient-dense, rightly portioned, and nutritionally compatible.

Through Optavia Fuelings, this may happen to many individuals; when you catch yourself losing weight, make sure to keep it smooth and steady. Pros and Cons of Optavia Diet

The Optavia diet depends on restrictive dinner substitution items and carefully calorie-controlled arranged suppers, so there's very little space for change.

The 5 and 1 plan limits calories to as low as 800-1000 every day, so it is not appropriate for women who are pregnant or individuals participating in an exercise that requires maximum physical activity.

Extraordinary calorie limitation can cause exhaustion, mind haze, cerebral pains, or menstrual changes. Al things considered, the 5 and 1 alternative ought not to be utilized long haul.

Be that as it May, the 3&3, and 4&2&1 Plan normally gracefully between 1100 to 2500 calories for every day and can be fitting to use for a more extended period.

After more than my 1-year journey in doing Optavia Diet, these are the following pros and cons I have noticed:

Pros:

Optavia's program may be a solid match for you on the off chance that you need a diet plan that is clear and simple to follow, that will assist you with getting in shape rapidly, and offers worked in social help.

Accomplishes Rapid Weight Loss

Most solid individuals require around 1600 to 3000 calories for each day to keep up their weight. Limiting that number to as low as 800 basically ensure weight loss for a great many people.

Optavia's 5&1 Plan is intended for brisk weight loss, making it a strong choice for somebody with a clinical motivation to shed pounds quickly.

You enter the fat-loss stage in just 3 days. Look for a Weight loss story on YouTube to see how many people out there are losing an impressing amount of weight, even 20 or more pounds in a week.

The average of 12 pounds in 12 weeks on the website counts all the people that do it by themselves, and nobody knows how many times they actually follow the plan, how many times they cheat, how much water they drink, exercise, etc.

Easy to Follow

As the diet depends on generally prepackaged Fuelings, you are only accountable for doing one meal a day on the 5&1 Plan.

Moreover, each individual plan comes with meal logs and a sample meal plan to make it easier for the client to follow.

Although you are encouraged to take 1 to 3 Lean and Green foods a day, contingent on the strategy, they are very simple to make—because the program will include detailed recipes and a list of food options for you to choose from.

In addition, those who are not keen on cooking can purchase prepackaged meals called Flavors of Home to substitute for the Lean and Green meals.

Bundled Items Offer Comfort

In spite of the fact that you should search for your own elements for "lean and green" dinners, the home conveyance choice for Optavia's "Fuelings" spares time and vitality.

When the items show up, they're anything but difficult to get ready and make phenomenal snatch and go suppers.

Packaged Products

They will be delivered directly at home, and they are quick-to-make and grab-and-go.

Social Support and Coaching

Stay motivated, do not cheat. Point out how people on coaching achieve a much faster and more massive weight loss.

Offers Social Help

Social help is a crucial part of achievement with any weight loss plan. Optavia's training project and gathering can give worked in consolation and backing for clients.

Optavia's health coaches are available throughout the weight loss and maintenance programs.

It's Not a Ketogenic Diet

Carbs are allowed and higher than the majority of weight-loss diets out there, just not the refined ones.

No Counting Calories

You don't really need to count your calories when following this type of diet, just as long as you stick with the rule of Fuelings, meals, snacks and water intake depending on your preference may it be 5&1, 4&2&1 or 3&3.

Cons

There are additionally some potential drawbacks to Optavia's plan, particularly on the off chance that you are stressed over cost, adaptability, and assortment.

It's Tough the First Weeks

You may feel hungry during the first weeks; however, it will fade away soon.

Low calories

Even though Optavia's diet plan emphasizes frequently eating throughout the day, each of its "Fuelings" only provides 110 calories. "Lean and Green" meals are also low in calories.

High Month-to-Month Cost

Optavia's expense can be an obstacle for imminent clients.

The 5&1 plan goes in cost from $350 to $425 for 119 servings (around three weeks of dinner substitutions).

Subsequent to picking your arrangement, you'll buy the food. Costs fluctuate and rely upon the amount you're purchasing (and what). It's frequently most straightforward to get one of their units. The Essential Optimal Kit, which sets with the 5&1 Optimal weight Plan, accompanies 119 portions of food (counting shakes, sides, soups, bars, snacks, sides, and pasta) for only $414.60. The Optimal Health Kit for the 3&3 Plan offers 130 food servings of comparative things for $333.

Weight Loss May Not Be Sustainable

One challenge familiar to anyone on a diet is determining how to maintain weight loss once they have completed the program.

May Be Incompatible with Other Eating Plans

The Optavia diet incorporates specific projects for veggie lovers, individuals with diabetes, and breastfeeding ladies. Moreover, around 66% of its items are affirmed sans gluten. In any case, alternatives are constrained for those on explicit diets.

For instance, Optavia Fuelings are not appropriate for veggie lovers or individuals with dairy hypersensitivities in light of the fact that most choices contain milk.

Moreover, the Fuelings utilize various fixings, so those with food hypersensitivities should peruse the names cautiously.

At long last, the Optavia program isn't suggested for pregnant ladies since it can't meet their dietary needs.

CHAPTER 6:

How Optavia Diet Can Help You Lose Weight

OPTAVIA diet plans are suitable for all persons regardless of current age or weight. However, such factors will determine how long you will continue using the diet plan. Current age, weight, and overall health will also determine how well a person conforms to the dietary program. The 2017 report funded by Medifast discovered that more than 70 percent of overweight adults who were placed on Medifast and received one-on-one behavioral support lost more than 5 percent of their body mass.

Following the Diet Plan

With the OPTAVIA diet plan, you will enjoy more than 60 Fueling options. However, you will find it difficult to stop going on that diet. Also, you would get to take in more Optavia meal every time without taking stock of what you are consuming. This is because there are no sugars, points, or calories to record.

More studies showed that sticking to the Optavia diet plan is easy compared to other regular eating regimens. According to a 2008 study published in the Diabetes Educator, 16 out of 119 Medifast dietitians completed the eating regimen in 86 weeks. In contrast, only eight out of the 119 participants that tried regular diets were able to continue for 86 weeks.

Recipes are available on different online platforms. Besides, it is possible to have a complete Optavia meal for dinner. It is fast and cheap to order meals and cook them. Adherents can also depend on their OPTAVIA instructors and online forums for knowledge and techniques.

The official Pinterest page of Optavia is an excellent example of where beginners can get some tips on the best lean and green meals. You can use the page as a conversion recipe guide to help you incorporate their ideas into your cooking plans.

Eating an all-out Optavia diet may be tough, but it is possible. The diet creators, Medifast group, recommend that you make a lean and green lunch for a day. There are tips and ideas on how to go about this on the company's official webpage. The guide available on the page offers tips for selecting drinks and picking toppings with condiments. For example, ask for your steak (not more than 7-ounce) to be provided without herbal butter and replace the baked potato with steamed broccoli.

Picking an eating regimen and making orders is very easy. Medifast group offers automatic delivery. The only difficulty that will be experienced when cooking OPTAVIA meals involves the addition of water and microwave nuking. Any random person or regular cook should be able to make a lean and green meal without much stress.

Medifast also states its diets have a healthy "fullness" level. This means that you can stay satisfied for a long time because of the high fiber and protein content. A 2010 report published in the Nutrition Journal observed that there are no significant discrepancies in satiety in post-meal or general fullness between the Optavia diet and other eating plans. The research on Diabetes Educator also found no significant association in dietary appetite across different types of diet. This is very important as specialists in nutrition have emphasized the relationship between satiety (the satisfying feeling you've had enough) and dietary plans.

Optavia diet from Medifast is ideal as the creators reveal that a panel tastes all their services before putting it on the market for their customers. The company also carries out different tracking of customer feedback regularly. Although this will not necessarily make the diet better than other dietary brands, the company believes it will satisfy their customers. OPTAVIA Fuelings do not involve artificial colors, sweeteners, or flavors.

CHAPTER 7:

Breakfast

1. Sun-Dried Tomato Garlic Bruschetta

Preparation Time: 10 minutes

Cooking Time: 5 minutes

Servings: 6

Ingredients:

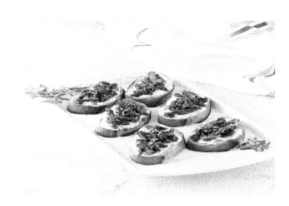

- 2 slices sourdough bread, toasted
- 1 tsp. chives, minced
- 1 garlic clove, peeled
- 2 tsp. sun-dried tomatoes in olive oil, minced
- 1 tsp. olive oil

Directions:

1. Vigorously rub garlic clove on 1 side of each of the toasted bread slices
2. Spread equal portions of sun-dried tomatoes on the garlic side of bread. Sprinkle chives and drizzle olive oil on top.
3. Pop both slices into oven toaster, and cook until well heated through.
4. Place bruschetta on a plate. Serve warm.

Nutrition:

Calories: 149 kcal

Protein: 6.12 g

Fat: 2.99 g

Carbohydrates: 24.39 g

2. Fantastic Spaghetti Squash with Cheese and Basil Pesto

Preparation Time: 10 minutes

Cooking Time: 35 minutes

Servings: 2

Ingredients:

- 1 cup cooked spaghetti squash, drained
- Salt, to taste
- Freshly cracked black pepper, to taste
- ½ tbsp. olive oil
- ¼ cup ricotta cheese, unsweetened
- 2oz fresh mozzarella cheese, cubed
- 1/8 cup basil pesto

Directions:

1. Switch on the oven, then set its temperature to 375 °F and let it preheat.
2. Meanwhile, take a medium bowl, add spaghetti squash in it and then season with salt and black pepper.
3. Take a casserole dish, grease it with oil, add squash mixture in it, top it with ricotta cheese and mozzarella cheese and bake for 10 minutes until cooked.
4. When done, remove the casserole dish from the oven, drizzle pesto on top and serve immediately.

Nutrition:

Calories 169

Total Fat 11.3g

Total Carbs 6.2g

Protein 11.9g

Sugar 0.1g

Sodium 217mg

3. Oat Porridge with Cherry & Coconut

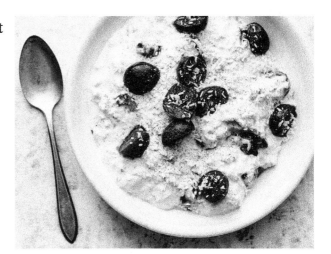

Preparation Time: 10 minutes

Cooking Time: 0 minutes

Servings: 3

Ingredients:

- 1 ½ cups regular oats
- 3 cups coconut milk
- 4 tbsp. chia seed
- 3 tbsp. raw cacao
- Coconut shavings
- Dark chocolate shavings
- Fresh or frozen tart cherries
- A pinch of stevia, optional
- Maple syrup, to taste (optional)

Directions:

1. Combine the oats, milk, stevia, and cacao in a medium saucepan over medium heat and bring to a boil. Lower the heat, then simmer until the oats are cooked to desired doneness.
2. Divide the porridge among 3 serving bowls and top with dark chocolate and coconut shavings, cherries, and a little drizzle of maple syrup.

Nutrition:

Calories: 343 kcal

Protein: 15.64 g

Fat: 12.78 g

Carbohydrates: 41.63 g

4. Gingerbread Oatmeal Breakfast

Preparation Time: 10 minutes

Cooking Time: 0 minutes

Servings: 4

Ingredients:

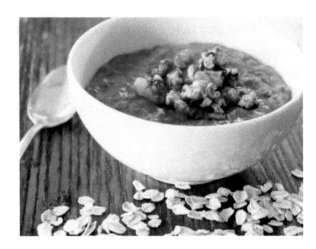

- 1 cup steel-cut oats
- 4 cups drinking water
- Organic Maple syrup, to taste
- 1 tsp ground cloves
- 1 ½ tbsp. ground cinnamon
- 1/8 tsp nutmeg
- ¼ tsp ground ginger
- ¼ tsp ground coriander
- ¼ tsp ground allspice
- ¼ tsp ground cardamom
- Fresh mixed berries

Directions:

1. Cook the oats based on the package instructions. When it comes to a boil, reduce heat and simmer.
2. Stir in all the spices and continue cooking until cooked to desired doneness.
3. Serve in four serving bowls and drizzle with maple syrup and top with fresh berries.
4. Enjoy!

Nutrition:

Calories: 87 kcal

Protein: 5.82 g

Fat: 3.26 g

Carbohydrates: 18.22 g

5. Breakfast Sausage and Mushroom Casserole

Preparation Time: 20 minutes

Cooking Time: 45 minutes

Servings: 4

Ingredients:

- 450g of Italian sausage, cooked and crumbled
- Three-fourth cup of coconut milk
- 8 ounces of white mushrooms, sliced
- 1 medium onion, finely diced
- 2 Tablespoons of organic ghee
- 6 free-range eggs
- 600g of sweet potatoes
- 1 red bell pepper, roasted
- 3/4 tsp. of ground black pepper, divided
- 1 ½ tsp. of sea salt, divided

Directions:

1. Peel and shred the sweet potatoes.
2. Take a bowl, fill it with ice-cold water, and soak the sweet potatoes in it. Set aside.
3. Peel the roasted bell pepper, remove its seeds and finely dice it.
4. Set the oven 375°F.
5. Get a casserole baking dish and grease it with the organic ghee.
6. Put a skillet over medium flame and cook the mushrooms in it. Cook until the mushrooms are crispy and brown.
7. Take the mushrooms out and mix them with the crumbled sausage.
8. Now sauté the onions in the same skillet. Cook up to the onions are soft and golden. This should take about 4 – 5 minutes.
9. Take the onions out and mix them in the sausage-mushroom mixture.
10. Add the diced bell pepper to the same mixture.
11. Mix well and set aside for a while.
12. Now drain the soaked shredded potatoes, put them on a paper towel, and pat dry.
13. Bring the sweet potatoes in a bowl and add about a teaspoon of salt and half a teaspoon of ground black pepper to it. Mix well and set aside.
14. Now take a large bowl and crack the eggs in it.
15. Break the eggs and then blend in the coconut milk.
16. Stir in the remaining black pepper and salt.
17. Take the greased casserole dish and spread the seasoned sweet potatoes evenly in the base of the dish. Next, spread the sausage mixture evenly in the dish.
18. Finally, spread the egg mixture. Now cover the casserole dish using a piece of aluminum foil.
19. Bake for 20 - 30 minutes. To check if the casserole is baked properly, insert a tester in the middle of the casserole, and it should come out clean.
20. Uncover the casserole dish and bake it again, uncovered for 5 - 10 minutes, until the casserole is a little golden on the top. Allow it to cool for 10 minutes.
21. Enjoy!

Nutrition:

Calories: 598 kcal Protein: 28.65 g Fat: 36.75 g Carbohydrates: 48.01 g

6. Yummy Steak Muffins

Preparation Time: 10 minutes

Cooking Time: 20 minutes

Servings: 4

Ingredients:

- 1 cup red bell pepper, diced
- 2 Tablespoons of water
- 8 ounce thin steak, cooked and finely chopped
- ¼ teaspoon of sea salt
- Dash of freshly ground black pepper
- 8 free-range eggs
- 1 cup of finely diced onion

Directions:

1. Set the oven to 350°F
2. Take 8 muffin tins and line then with parchment paper liners.
3. Get a large bowl and crack all the eggs in it.
4. Beat well the eggs.
5. Blend in all the remaining ingredients.
6. Spoon the batter into the arrange muffin tins. Fill three-fourth of each tin.
7. Put the muffin tins in the preheated oven for about 20 minutes, until the muffins are baked and set in the middle.
8. Enjoy!

Nutrition:

Calories: 151 kcal

Protein: 17.92 g

Fat: 7.32 g

Carbohydrates: 3.75 g

7. Banana Cashew Toast

Preparation Time: 10 minutes

Cooking Time: 0 minutes

Servings: 3

Ingredients:

- 1 cup roasted cashews (unsalted)
- 4 pieces oat bread
- 2 ripe medium-sized bananas
- Dash of salt
- Pinch of cinnamon
- 2 tsp. flax meals
- 2 tsp. honey

Directions:

1. Peel and slice the bananas into ½-inch pieces. Toast the bread. In a food processor, puree the salt and cashews until they are smooth. Use the puree as a spread on the toasts. On top of the spread, arrange a layer of bananas. Add flax meals and a dash of cinnamon on top of the bananas. Top the toast with honey.

Nutrition:

Calories: 634 kcal

Protein: 13.42 g

Fat: 47.6 g

Carbohydrates: 48.02 g

8. Hash Browns

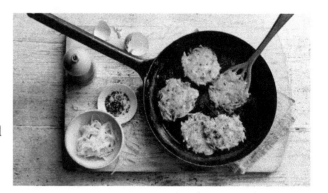

Preparation Time: 15 minutes

Cooking Time: 15 minutes

Servings: 4

Ingredients:

- 1 pound Russet potatoes, peeled, processed using a grater
- Pinch of sea salt
- Pinch of black pepper, to taste
- 3 Tbsp. olive oil

Directions:

1. Line a microwave safe-dish with paper towels. Spread shredded potatoes on top. Microwave veggies on the highest heat setting for 2 minutes. Remove from heat.
2. Pour 1 tablespoon of oil into a non-stick skillet set over medium heat.
3. Cooking in batches, place a generous pinch of potatoes into the hot oil. Press down using the back of a spatula.
4. Cook for 3 minutes every side, or until brown and crispy. Drain on paper towels. Repeat step for remaining potatoes. Add more oil as needed.
5. Season with salt and pepper. Serve.

Nutrition:

Calories:

200 kcal

Protein: 4.03 g

Fat: 11.73 g

Carbohydrates: 20.49 g

9. White and Green Quiche

Preparation Time: 10 minutes

Cooking Time: 40 minutes

Servings: 3

Ingredients:

- 3 cups of fresh spinach, chopped
- 15 large free-range eggs
- 3 cloves of garlic, minced
- 5 white mushrooms, sliced
- 1 small sized onion, finely chopped
- 1 ½ teaspoon of baking powder
- Ground black pepper to taste
- 1 ½ cups of coconut milk
- Ghee, as required to grease the dish
- Sea salt to taste

Directions:

1. Set the oven to 350°F.
2. Get a baking dish then grease it with the organic ghee.
3. Break all the eggs in a huge bowl then whisk well.
4. Stir in coconut milk. Beat well
5. While you are whisking the eggs, start adding the remaining ingredients in it.
6. When all the ingredients are thoroughly blended, pour all of it into the prepared baking dish.
7. Bake for at least 40 minutes, up to the quiche is set in the middle.
8. Enjoy!

Nutrition:

Calories: 608 kcal

Protein: 20.28 g

Fat: 53.42 g

Carbohydrates: 16.88 g

10. Beef Breakfast Casserole

Preparation Time: 10 minutes

Cooking Time: 30 minutes

Servings: 5

Ingredients:

- 1 pound of ground beef, cooked
- 10 eggs
- ½ cup Pico de Gallo
- 1 cup baby spinach
- ¼ cup sliced black olives
- Freshly ground black pepper

Directions:

1. Preheat oven to 350 degrees Fahrenheit. Prepare a 9" glass pie plate with non-stick spray.
2. Whisk the eggs until frothy. Season with salt and pepper.
3. Layer the cooked ground beef, Pico de Gallo, and spinach in the pie plate.
4. Slowly pour the eggs over the top.
5. Top with black olives.
6. Bake for at least 30 minutes, until firm in the middle.
7. Slice into 5 pieces and serve.

Nutrition:

Calories: 479 kcal Protein: 43.54 g Fat: 30.59 g Carbohydrates: 4.65 g

11. Tomato and Avocado Omelet

Preparation Time: 5 minutes

Cooking Time: 5 minutes

Servings: 1

Ingredients:

- 2 eggs
- ¼ avocado, diced
- 4 cherry tomatoes, halved
- 1 tablespoon cilantro, chopped
- Squeeze of lime juice
- Pinch of salt

Directions:

1. Put together the avocado, tomatoes, cilantro, lime juice, and salt in a small bowl, then mix well and set aside.
2. Warm a medium nonstick skillet on medium heat. Whisk the eggs until frothy and add to the pan. Move the eggs around gently with a rubber spatula until they begin to set.
3. Scatter the avocado mixture over half of the omelet. Remove from heat, and slide the omelet onto a plate as you fold it in half.
4. Serve immediately.

Nutrition:

Calories: 433 kcal Protein: 25.55 g Fat: 32.75 g Carbohydrates: 10.06 g

12. Mango Granola

Preparation Time: 10 minutes
Cooking Time: 30 minutes
Servings: 4
Ingredients:

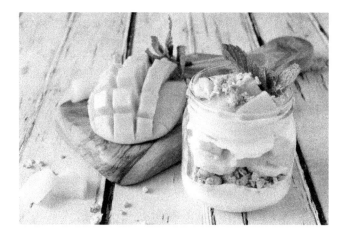

- 2 cups rolled oats
- 1 cup dried mango, chopped
- ½ cup almonds, roughly chopped
- ½ cup nuts
- ½ cup dates, roughly chopped
- 3 tbsp. sesame seeds
- 2 tsp. cinnamon
- 2/3 cup agave nectar
- 2 tbsp. coconut oil
- 2 tbsp. water

Directions:

1. Set oven at 320F
2. In a large bowl, put the oats, almonds, nuts, sesame seeds, dates, and cinnamon then mix well.
3. Meanwhile, heat a saucepan over medium heat, pour in the agave syrup, coconut oil, and water.
4. Stir and let it cook for at least 3 minutes or until the coconut oil has melted.
5. Gradually pour the syrup mixture into the bowl with the oats and nuts and stir well, ensure that all the ingredients are coated with the syrup.
6. Transfer the granola on a baking sheet lined with parchment paper and place in the oven to bake for 20 minutes.
7. After 20 minutes, take off the tray from the oven and lay the chopped dried mango on top. Put back in the oven then bake again for another 5 minutes.
8. Let the granola cool to room temperature before serving or placing it in an airtight container for storage. The shelf life of the granola will last up to 2-3 weeks.

Nutrition:

Calories: 434 kcal

Protein: 13.16 g

Fat: 28.3 g

Carbohydrates: 55.19 g

13. Cheesy Flax and Hemp Seeds Muffins

Preparation Time: 5 minutes

Cooking Time: 30 minutes

Servings: 2

Ingredients:

- 1/8 cup flax seeds meal
- ¼ cup raw hemp seeds
- ¼ cup almond meal
- Salt, to taste
- ¼ tsp baking powder
- 3 organic eggs, beaten
- 1/8 cup nutritional yeast flakes
- ¼ cup cottage cheese, low-fat
- ¼ cup grated parmesan cheese
- ¼ cup scallion, sliced thinly
- 1 tbsp. olive oil

Directions:

1. Switch on the oven, then set it 360°F and let it preheat.
2. Meanwhile, take two ramekins, grease them with oil, and set aside until required.
3. Take a medium bowl, add flax seeds, hemp seeds, and almond meal, and then stir in salt and baking powder until mixed.
4. Crack eggs in another bowl, add yeast, cottage cheese, and parmesan, stir well until combined, and then stir this mixture into the almond meal mixture until incorporated.
5. Fold in scallions, then distribute the mixture between prepared ramekins and bake for 30 minutes until muffins are firm and the top is nicely golden brown.
6. When done, take out the muffins from the ramekins and let them cool completely on a wire rack.
7. For meal prepping, wrap each muffin with a paper towel and refrigerate for up to thirty-four days.
8. When ready to eat, reheat muffins in the microwave until hot and then serve.

Nutrition:

Calories 179

Total Fat 10.9g

Total Carbs 6.9g

Protein 15.4g

Sugar 2.3g

Sodium 311mg

14. Flaxseed Porridge with Cinnamon

Preparation Time: 10 minutes

Cooking Time: 5 minutes

Servings: 4

Ingredients:

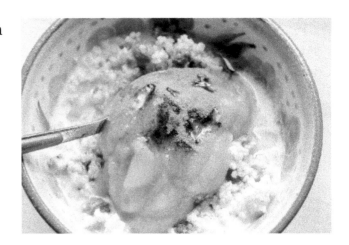

- 1 tsp cinnamon
- 1½ tsp stevia
- 1 tbsp. unsalted butter
- 2 tbsp. flaxseed meal
- 2 tbsp. flaxseed oatmeal
- ½ cup shredded coconut
- 1 cup heavy cream
- 2 cups of water

Directions:

1. Take a medium pot, place it over low heat, add all the ingredients in it, stir until mixed and bring the mixture to boil.
2. When the mixture has boiled, remove the pot from heat, stir it well and divide it evenly between four bowls.
3. Let porridge rest for 10 minutes until slightly thicken and then serve.

Nutrition:

Calories 171

Total Fat 16g

Total Carbs 6g

Protein 2g

15. Anti-Inflammatory Breakfast Frittata

Preparation Time: 10 minutes

Cooking Time: 40 minutes

Servings: 4

Ingredients:

- 4 large eggs
- 6 egg whites
- 450g button mushrooms
- 450g baby spinach
- 125g firm tofu
- 1 onion, chopped
- 1 tbsp. minced garlic
- ½ tsp. ground turmeric
- ½ tsp. cracked black pepper
- ¼ cup water
- Kosher salt to taste

Directions:

1. Set your oven to 350F.
2. Sauté the mushrooms in a little bit of extra virgin olive oil in a large non-stick ovenproof pan over medium heat. Add the onions once the mushrooms start turning golden and cook for 3 minutes until the onions become soft.
3. Stir in the garlic then cook for at least 30 seconds until fragrant before adding the spinach. Pour in water, cover, and cook until the spinach becomes wilted for about 2 minutes.
4. Take off the lid and continue cooking up to the water evaporates. Now, combine the eggs, egg whites, tofu, pepper, turmeric, and salt in a bowl. When all the liquid has evaporated, pour in the egg mixture, let cook for about 2 minutes until the edges start setting, then transfer to the oven and bake for about 25 minutes or until cooked.
5. Take off from the oven then let sit for at least 5 minutes before cutting it into quarters and serving.
6. Enjoy!
7. Baby spinach and mushrooms boost the nutrient profile of the eggs to provide you with amazing anti-inflammatory benefits.

Nutrition:

Calories: 521 kcal

Protein: 29.13 g

Fat: 10.45 g

Carbohydrates: 94.94 g

16. Shirataki Pasta with Avocado and Cream

Preparation Time: 10 minutes

Cooking Time: 6 minutes

Servings: 2

Ingredients:

- ½ packet of shirataki noodles, cooked
- ½ of an avocado
- ½ tsp cracked black pepper
- ½ tsp salt
- ½ tsp dried basil
- 1/8 cup heavy cream

Directions:

1. Place a medium pot half full with water over medium heat, bring it to boil, then add noodles and cook for 2 minutes.
2. Then drain the noodles and set aside until required.
3. Place avocado in a bowl, mash it with a fork,
4. Mash avocado in a bowl, transfer it in a blender, add remaining ingredients, and pulse until smooth.
5. Take a frying pan, place it over medium heat and when hot, add noodles in it, pour in the avocado mixture, stir well and cook for 2 minutes until hot.
6. Serve straight away.

Nutrition:

Calories 131 Total Fat 12.6g Total Carbs 4.9g Protein 1.2g Sugar 0.3g Sodium 588mg

17. Apple Oatmeal

Preparation Time: 10 minutes

Cooking Time: 5 minutes

Servings: 2

Ingredients:

- 2/3 cups rolled oats
- 1 cup water
- 1 teaspoon ground cinnamon
- 1 cup of any non-fat milk, coconut milk or almond milk (optional)
- ¼ cup fresh apple juice
- 1 chopped apple, (unpeeled or peeled)

Directions:

1. Place the water, juice, and the apple in a deep pot. Bring to boil over medium heat.
2. Add the oats and cinnamon. Bring to another boil. Lower the heat temperature and let it simmer for 3 minutes or until it is thick.
3. Divide the serving into two and serve with milk.

Nutrition:

Calories: 277 kcal Protein: 12.69 g Fat: 7.69 g Carbohydrates: 52.71 g

CHAPTER 8:

Lunch

18. Optavia Pizza Hack

Preparation Time: 5-10 minutes
Cooking Time: 15-20 minutes
Servings: 1
Ingredients:

- 1/4 fueling of garlic mashed potato
- 1/2 egg whites
- 1/4 tablespoon of baking powder
- 3/4 oz. of reduced-fat shredded mozzarella
- 1/8 cup of sliced white mushrooms
- 1/16 cup of pizza sauce
- 3/4 oz. of ground beef
- 1/4 sliced black olives
- You also need a sauté pan, baking sheets, and parchment paper

Directions:

1. Start by preheating the oven to 400°.
2. Mix your baking powder and garlic potato packet.
3. Add egg whites to your mixture and stir well until it blends.
4. Line the baking sheet with parchment paper and pour the mixed batter onto it.
5. Put another parchment paper on top of the batter and spread out the batter to a 1/8-inch circle.
6. Then place another baking sheet on top; this way, the batter is between two baking sheets.
7. Place into an oven and bake for about 8 minutes until the pizza crust is golden brown.
8. For the toppings, place your ground beef in a sauté pan and fry till it's brown and wash your mushrooms very well.
9. After the crust is baked, remove the top layer of parchment paper carefully to prevent the foam from sticking to the pizza crust.
10. Put your toppings on top of the crust and bake for an extra 8 minutes.
11. Once ready, slide the pizza off the parchment paper and onto a plate.

Nutrition:
Calories: 478
Protein: 30 g
Carbohydrates: 22 g
Fats: 29 g

19. Amaranth Porridge

Preparation Time: 5 minutes
Cooking Time: 30 minutes
Servings: 2.
Ingredients:

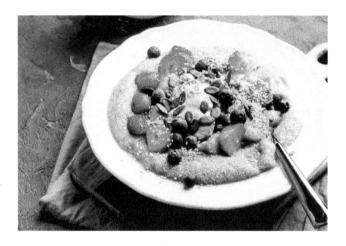

- 2 cups coconut milk
- 2 cups alkaline water
- 1 cup amaranth
- 2 tbsps. coconut oil
- 1 tbsp. ground cinnamon

Directions:

1. In a saucepan, mix in the milk with water, then boil the mixture.
2. You stir in the amaranth, then reduce the heat to medium.
3. Cook on the medium heat, then simmer for at least 30 minutes as you stir it occasionally.
4. Turn off the heat.
5. Add in cinnamon and coconut oil then stir.
6. Serve.

Nutrition:

Calories: 434 kcal

Fat: 35g

Carbs: 27g

Protein: 6.7g

20. Gluten-Free Pancakes

Preparation Time: 5 minutes

Cooking Time: 2 minutes

Servings: 2

Ingredients:

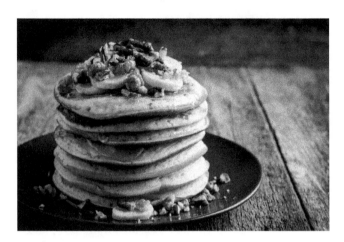

- 6 eggs
- 1 cup low-fat cream cheese
- 1 1/12; teaspoons baking powder
- 1 scoop protein powder
- 1/4 cup almond meal
- ¼ teaspoon salt

Directions:

1. Combine dry ingredients in a food processor. Add the eggs one after another and then the cream cheese. Mix it well.
2. Lightly grease a skillet with cooking spray and place over medium-high heat.
3. Pour the batter into the pan. Turn the pan gently to create round pancakes.
4. Cook for about 2 minutes on each side.
5. Serve pancakes with your favorite topping.

Nutrition:

Dietary Fiber: 1 g

Net Carbs: 5 g

Protein: 25 g

Total Fat: 14 g

Calories: 288

21. Mushroom & Spinach Omelet

Preparation Time: 20 minutes

Cooking Time: 20 minutes

Servings: 3

Ingredients:

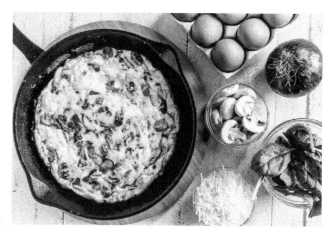

- 2 tablespoons butter, divided
- 6-8 fresh mushrooms, sliced, 5 ounces
- Chives, chopped, optional
- Salt and pepper, to taste
- 1 handful baby spinach, about 1/2 ounce
- Pinch garlic powder
- 4 eggs, beaten
- 1-ounce shredded Swiss cheese

Directions:

1. In a very large saucepan, sauté the mushrooms in one tablespoon of butter until soft. Season with salt, pepper, and garlic.

2. Remove the mushrooms from the pan and keep warm. Heat the remaining tablespoon of butter in the same skillet over medium heat.

3. Beat the eggs with a little salt and pepper and add to the hot butter. Turn the pan over to coat the entire bottom of the pan with egg. Once the egg is almost out, place the cheese over the middle of the tortilla.

4. Fill the cheese with spinach leaves and hot mushrooms. Let cook for about a minute for the spinach to start to wilt. Fold the empty side of the tortilla carefully over the filling and slide it onto a plate and sprinkle with chives, if desired.

5. Alternatively, you can make two tortillas using half the mushroom, spinach, and cheese filling in each.

Nutrition:

Calories: 321 Fat: 26 g

Protein: 19 g Carbohydrate: 4 g

Dietary Fiber: 1 g

22. Sweet Cashew Cheese Spread

Preparation Time: 5 minutes
Cooking Time: 5 minutes
Servings: 10 servings
Ingredients:

- Stevia (5 drops)
- Cashews (2 cups, raw)
- Water (1/2 cup)

Directions:

1. Soak the cashews overnight in water.
2. Next, drain the excess water then transfer cashews to a food processor.
3. Add in the stevia and the water.
4. Process until smooth.
5. **Serve chilled. Enjoy.**

Nutrition:

Fat: 7 g
Cholesterol: 0 mg
Sodium: 12.6 mg
Carbohydrates: 5.7 g

23. Mini Zucchini Bites

Preparation Time: 10 minutes
Cooking Time: 10 minutes
Servings: 6
Ingredients:

- 1 zucchini, cut into thick circles
- 3 cherry tomatoes, halved
- 1/2 cup parmesan cheese, grated
- Salt and pepper to taste
- 1 tsp. chives, chopped

Directions:

1. Preheat the oven to 390 degrees F.
2. Add wax paper on a baking sheet.
3. Arrange the zucchini pieces.
4. Add the cherry halves on each zucchini slice.
5. Add parmesan cheese, chives, and sprinkle with salt and pepper.
6. Bake for 10 minutes. Serve.

Nutrition:

Fat: 1.0 g Cholesterol: 5.0 mg Sodium: 400.3 mg Potassium: 50.5 mg Carbohydrates: 7.3 g

24. Hemp Seed Porridge

Preparation Time: 5 minutes

Cooking Time: 5 minutes

Servings: 6

Ingredients:

- 3 cups cooked hemp seed
- 1 packet Stevia
- 1 cup coconut milk

Directions:

1. In a saucepan, mix the rice and the coconut milk over moderate heat for about 5 minutes as you stir it constantly.
2. Remove the pan from the burner then add the Stevia. Stir.
3. Serve in 6 bowls.
4. Enjoy.

Nutrition:

Calories: 236 kcal

Fat: 1.8 g

Carbs: 48.3 g

Protein: 7 g

25. Mini Mac in a Bowl

Preparation Time: 5 minutes

Cooking Time: 15 minutes

Servings: 1

Ingredients:

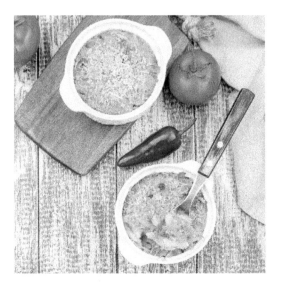

- 5 ounces of lean ground beef
- Two tablespoons of diced white or yellow onion.
- 1/8 teaspoon of onion powder
- 1/8 teaspoon of white vinegar
- 1 ounce of dill pickle slices
- One teaspoon sesame seed
- 3 cups of shredded Romaine lettuce
- Cooking spray
- Two tablespoons reduced-fat shredded cheddar cheese
- Two tablespoons of Wish-Bone light thousand island as dressing

Directions:

1. Place a lightly greased small skillet on fire to heat.
2. Add your onion to cook for about 2-3 minutes.
3. Next, add the beef and allow cooking until it's brown.
4. Next, mix your vinegar and onion powder with the dressing.
5. Finally, top the lettuce with the cooked meat and sprinkle cheese on it, add your pickle slices.
6. Drizzle the mixture with the sauce and sprinkle the sesame seeds.
7. Your mini mac in a bowl is ready for consumption.

Nutrition:

Calories: 150

Protein: 21 g

Carbohydrates: 32 g

Fats: 19 g

26. Shake Cake Fueling

Preparation Time: 5 minutes

Cooking Time: 0 minutes

Servings: 1

Ingredients:

- One packet of Optavia shakes.
- 1/4 teaspoon of baking powder
- Two tablespoons of eggbeaters or egg whites
- Two tablespoons of water
- Other options that are not compulsory include sweetener, reduced-fat cream cheese, etc.

Directions:

1. Begin by preheating the oven.
2. Mix all the ingredients. Begin with the dry ingredients, and then add the wet ingredients.
3. After the mixture/batter is ready, pour gently into muffin cups.
4. Inside the oven, place, and bake for about 16-18 minutes or until it is baked and ready. Allow it to cool completely.
5. Add additional toppings of your choice and ensure your delicious shake cake is refreshing.

Nutrition:

Calories: 896 Fat: 37 g Carbohydrate: 115 g Protein: 34 g

27. Optavia Biscuit Pizza

Preparation Time: 5 minutes

Cooking Time: 15-20 minutes

Servings: 1

Ingredients:

- 1/4 sachet of Optavia buttermilk cheddar and herb biscuit
- 1/4 tablespoon of tomato sauce
- 1/4 tablespoon of low-fat shredded cheese
- ¼ bottle of water
- Parchment paper

Directions:

1. Begin by preheating the oven to about 350°F
2. Mix the biscuit and water and stir properly.
3. In the parchment paper, pour the mixture and spread it into a thin circle. Allow cooking for 10 minutes.
4. Take it out and add the tomato sauce and shredded cheese.
5. Bake it for a few more minutes.

Nutrition:

Calories: 478 Protein: 30 g Carbohydrates: 22 g Fats: 29 g

28. Lean and Green Smoothie 1

Preparation Time: 5 minutes
Cooking Time: 0 minutes
Servings: 1
Ingredients:

- 2 1/2 cups of kale leaves
- 3/4 cup of chilled apple juice
- 1 cup of cubed pineapple
- 1/2 cup of frozen green grapes
- 1/2 cup of chopped apple

Directions:

1. Place the pineapple, apple juice, apple, frozen seedless grapes, and kale leaves in a blender.
2. Cover and blend until it's smooth.
3. Smoothie is ready and can be garnished with halved grapes if you wish.

Nutrition:

Calories: 81
Protein: 2 g
Carbohydrates: 19 g
Fats: 1 g

29. Lean and Green Smoothie 2

Preparation Time: 5 minutes
Cooking Time: 0 minutes
Servings: 1
Ingredients:

- Six kale leaves
- Two peeled oranges
- 2 cups of mango kombucha
- 2 cups of chopped pineapple
- 2 cups of water

Directions:

1. Break up the oranges, place in the blender.
2. Add the mango kombucha, chopped pineapple, and kale leaves into the blender.
3. Blend everything until it is smooth.
4. Smoothie is ready to be taken.

Nutrition:

Calories: 81 Protein: 2 g Carbohydrates: 19 g Fats: 1 g

30. Lean and Green Chicken Pesto Pasta

Preparation Time: 5 minutes

Cooking Time: 15 minutes

Servings: 1

Ingredients:

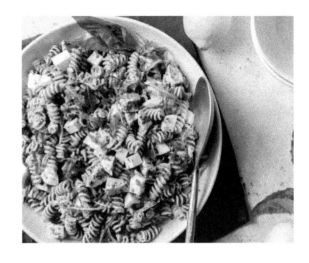

- 3 cups of raw kale leaves
- 2 tbsp. of olive oil
- 2 cups of fresh basil
- 1/4 teaspoon salt
- 3 tbsp. lemon juice
- Three garlic cloves
- 2 cups of cooked chicken breast
- 1 cup of baby spinach
- 6 ounces of uncooked chicken pasta
- 3 ounces of diced fresh mozzarella
- Basil leaves or red pepper flakes to garnish

Directions:

1. Start by making the pesto; add the kale, lemon juice, basil, garlic cloves, olive oil, and salt to a blender and blend until its smooth.
2. Add salt and pepper to taste.
3. Cook the pasta and strain off the water. Reserve 1/4 cup of the liquid.
4. Get a bowl and mix everything, the cooked pasta, pesto, diced chicken, spinach, mozzarella, and the reserved pasta liquid.
5. Sprinkle the mixture with additional chopped basil or red paper flakes (optional).
6. Now your salad is ready. You may serve it warm or chilled. Also, it can be taken as a salad mix-ins or as a side dish. Leftovers should be stored in the refrigerator inside an air-tight container for 3-5 days.

Nutrition:

Calories: 244

Protein: 20.5 g

Carbohydrates: 22.5 g

Fats: 10 g

31. Open-Face Egg Sandwiches with Cilantro-Jalapeño Spread

Preparation Time: 20 minutes

Cooking Time: 10 minutes

Servings: 2

Ingredients:

For the cilantro and jalapeño spread

- 1 cup filled up fresh cilantro leaves and stems (about a bunch)
- 1 jalapeño pepper, seeded and roughly chopped
- ½ cup extra-virgin olive oil
- ¼ cup pepitas (hulled pumpkin seeds), raw or roasted
- 2 garlic cloves, thinly sliced
- 1 tablespoon freshly squeezed lime juice
- 1 teaspoon kosher salt

For the eggs

- 4 large eggs
- ¼ cup milk
- ¼ to ½ teaspoon kosher salt
- 2 tablespoons butter

For the sandwich

- 2 slices bread
- 1 tablespoon butter
- 1 avocado, halved, pitted, and divided into slices
- Microgreens or sprouts, for garnish

Directions:

To make the cilantro and jalapeño spread

1. In a food processor, combine the cilantro, jalapeño, oil, pepitas, garlic, lime juice, and salt. Whirl until smooth. Refrigerate if making in advance; otherwise set aside.

To make the eggs

2. In a medium bowl, whisk the eggs, milk, and salt.
3. Dissolve the butter in a skillet over low heat, swirling to coat the bottom of the pan. Pour in the whisked eggs.
4. Cook until they begin to set then, using a heatproof spatula, push them to the sides, allowing the uncooked portions to run into the bottom of the skillet.
5. Continue until the eggs are set.

To assemble the sandwiches

1. Toast the bed and spread with butter.
2. Spread a spoonful of the cilantro-jalapeño spread on each piece of toast. Top each with scrambled eggs. Arrange avocado over each sandwich and garnish with microgreens.

Nutrition:

Calories: 711 Total fat: 4 g Cholesterol: 54 mg Fiber: 12 g Protein: 12 g Sodium: 327 mg

CHAPTER 9:

Lunch

32. Crunchy Quinoa Meal

Preparation Time: 5 minutes
Cooking Time: 25 minutes
Servings: 2
Ingredients:

- 3 cups coconut milk
- 1 cup rinsed quinoa
- 1/8 tsp. ground cinnamon
- 1 cup raspberry
- 1/2 cup chopped coconuts

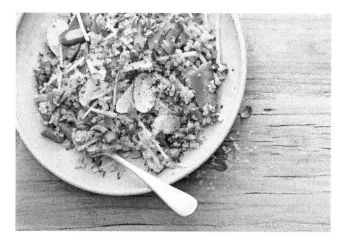

Directions:

1. In a saucepan, pour milk and bring to a boil over moderate heat.
2. Add the quinoa to the milk and then bring it to a boil once more.
3. You then let it simmer for at least 15 minutes on medium heat until the milk is reduced.
4. Stir in the cinnamon then mix properly.
5. Cover it then cook for 8 minutes until the milk is completely absorbed.
6. Add the raspberry and cook the meal for 30 seconds.
7. Serve and enjoy.

Nutrition:

Calories: 271 kcal

Fat: 3.7g

Carbs: 54g

Proteins: 6.5g

33. Quinoa Porridge

Preparation Time: 5 minutes

Cooking Time: 25 minutes

Servings: 2

Ingredients:

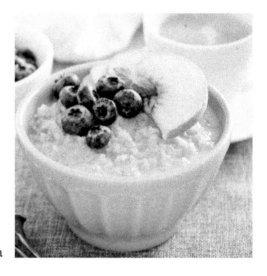

- 2 cups coconut milk
- 1 cup rinsed quinoa
- 1/8 tsp. ground cinnamon
- 1 cup fresh blueberries

Directions:

1. In a saucepan, boil the coconut milk over high heat.
2. Add the quinoa to the milk then bring the mixture to a boil.
3. You then let it simmer for 15 minutes on medium heat until the milk is reduces.
4. Add the cinnamon then mix it properly in the saucepan.
5. Cover the saucepan and cook for at least 8 minutes until milk is completely absorbed.
6. Add in the blueberries then cook for 30 more seconds.
7. Serve.

Nutrition:

Calories: 271 kcal

Fat: 3.7g

Carbs: 54g

Protein: 6.5g

34. Banana Barley Porridge

Preparation Time: 15 minutes

Cooking Time: 5 minutes

Servings: 2

Ingredients:

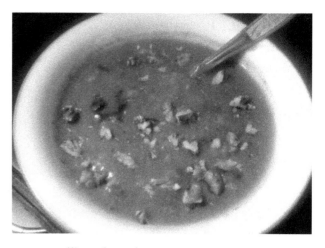

- 1 cup divided unsweetened coconut milk
- 1 small peeled and sliced banana
- 1/2 cup barley
- 3 drops liquid stevia
- 1/4 cup chopped coconuts

Directions:

1. In a bowl, properly mix barley with half of the coconut milk and stevia.
2. Cover the mixing bowl then refrigerate for about 6 hours.
3. In a saucepan, mix the barley mixture with coconut milk.
4. Cook for about 5 minutes on moderate heat.
5. Then top it with the chopped coconuts and the banana slices.
6. Serve.

Nutrition:

Calories: 159kcal

Fat: 8.4g

Carbs: 19.8g

Proteins: 4.6g

35. Millet Porridge

Preparation Time: 10 minutes
Cooking Time: 20 minutes
Servings: 2
Ingredients:

- Sea salt
- 1 tbsp. finely chopped coconuts
- 1/2 cup unsweetened coconut milk
- 1/2 cup rinsed and drained millet
- 1-1/2 cups alkaline water
- 3 drops liquid stevia

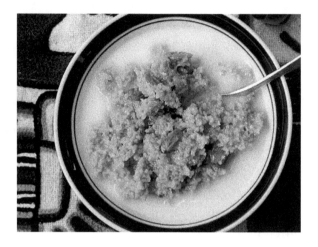

Directions:

1. Sauté the millet in a non-stick skillet for about 3 minutes.
2. Add salt and water then stir.
3. Let the meal boil then reduce the amount of heat.
4. Cook for 15 minutes then add the remaining ingredients. Stir.
5. Cook the meal for 4 extra minutes.
6. Serve the meal with toping of the chopped nuts.

Nutrition:

Calories: 219 kcal

Fat: 4.5g

Carbs: 38.2g

Protein: 6.4g

36. Jackfruit Vegetable Fry

Preparation Time: 5 minutes

Cooking Time: 5 minutes

Servings: 6

Ingredients:

- 2 finely chopped small onions
- 2 cups finely chopped cherry tomatoes
- 1/8 tsp. ground turmeric
- 1 tbsp. olive oil
- 2 seeded and chopped red bell peppers
- 3 cups seeded and chopped firm jackfruit
- 1/8 tsp. cayenne pepper
- 2 tbsps. chopped fresh basil leaves
- Salt

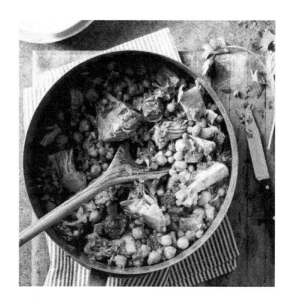

Directions:

1. In a greased skillet, sauté the onions and bell peppers for about 5 minutes.
2. Add the tomatoes then stir.
3. Cook for 2 minutes.
4. Then add the jackfruit, cayenne pepper, salt, and turmeric.
5. Cook for about 8 minutes.
6. Garnish the meal with basil leaves.
7. Serve warm.

Nutrition:

Calories: 236 kcal

Fat: 1.8g

Carbs: 48.3g

Protein: 7g

37. Zucchini Pancakes

Preparation Time: 15 minutes

Cooking Time: 8 minutes

Servings: 8

Ingredients:

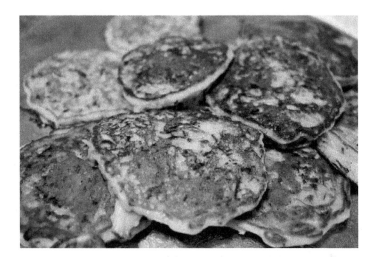

- 12 tbsps. alkaline water
- 6 large grated zucchinis
- Sea salt
- 4 tbsps. ground Flax Seeds
- 2 tsps. olive oil
- 2 finely chopped jalapeño peppers
- 1/2 cup finely chopped scallions

Directions:

1. In a bowl, mix together water and the flax seeds then set it aside.
2. Pour oil in a large non-stick skillet then heat it on medium heat.
3. Then add the black pepper, salt, and zucchini.
4. Cook for 3 minutes then transfer the zucchini into a large bowl.
5. Add the flax seed and the scallion's mixture then properly mix it.
6. Preheat a griddle then grease it lightly with the cooking spray.
7. Pour 1/4 of the zucchini mixture into griddle then cook for 3 minutes.
8. Flip the side carefully then cook for 2 more minutes.
9. Repeat the procedure with the remaining mixture in batches.
10. Serve.

Nutrition:

Calories: 71 kcal

Fat: 2.8g

Carbs: 9.8g

Protein: 3.7g

38. Squash Hash

Preparation Time: 2 minutes
Cooking Time: 10 minutes
Servings: 2
Ingredients:

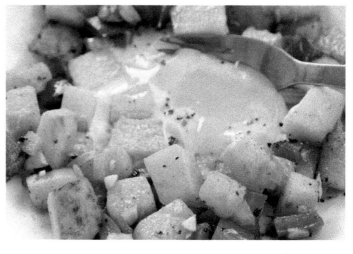

- 1 tsp. onion powder
- 1/2 cup finely chopped onion
- 2 cups spaghetti squash
- 1/2 tsp. sea salt

Directions:

1. Using paper towels, squeeze extra moisture from spaghetti squash.
2. Place the squash into a bowl then add the salt, onion, and the onion powder.
3. Stir properly to mix them.
4. Spray a non-stick cooking skillet with cooking spray then place it over moderate heat.
5. Add the spaghetti squash to pan.
6. Cook the squash for about 5 minutes.
7. Flip the hash browns using a spatula.
8. Cook for 5 minutes until the desired crispness is reached.
9. Serve.

Nutrition:

Calories: 44 kcal

Fat: 0.6g

Carbs: 9.7g

Protein: 0.9g

39. Pumpkin Spice Quinoa

Preparation Time: 10 minutes

Cooking Time: 0 minutes

Servings: 2

Ingredients:

- 1 cup cooked quinoa
- 1 cup unsweetened coconut milk
- 1 large mashed banana
- 1/4 cup pumpkin puree
- 1 tsp. pumpkin spice
- 2 tsps. chia seeds

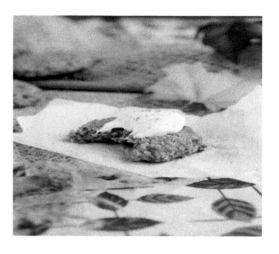

Directions:

1. In a container, mix all the ingredients.
2. Seal the lid then shake the container properly to mix.
3. Refrigerate overnight.
4. Serve.

Nutrition:

Calories: 212 kcal

Fat: 11.9g

Carbs: 31.7g

Protein: 7.3g

40. Cheesy Spicy Bacon Bowls

Preparation Time: 10 minutes

Cooking Time: 22 minutes

Servings: 12

Ingredients:

- 6 strips Bacon, pan-fried until cooked but still malleable
- 4 eggs
- 60 grams' cheddar cheese
- 40 grams' cream cheese, grated
- 2 Jalapenos, sliced and seeds removed
- 2 tablespoons coconut oil
- ¼ teaspoon onion powder
- ¼ teaspoon garlic powder
- Dash of salt and pepper

Directions:

1. Preheat oven to 375 degrees Fahrenheit
2. In a bowl, beat together eggs, cream cheese, jalapenos (minus 6 slices), coconut oil, onion powder, garlic powder, and salt and pepper.
3. Using leftover bacon grease on a muffin tray, rubbing it into each insert. Place bacon-wrapped inside the parameters of each insert.
4. Pour beaten mixture halfway up each bacon bowl.
5. Garnish each bacon bowl with cheese and leftover jalapeno slices (placing one on top of each).
6. Leave in the oven for about 22 minutes, or until the egg is thoroughly cooked and cheese is bubbly.
7. Remove from oven and let cool until edible.
8. Enjoy!

Nutrition:

Calories: 259
Fat: 24g
Carbs: 1g
Fiber: 0g
Protein: 10g

41. Goat, Cheese, Zucchini, and Kale Quiche

Preparation Time: 35 minutes
Cooking Time: 1 hour 10 minutes
Servings: 4
Ingredients:

- 4 large eggs
- 8 ounces fresh zucchini, sliced
- 10 ounces kale
- 3 garlic cloves (minced)
- 1 cup of soy milk
- 1-ounce goat cheese
- 1 cup grated parmesan
- 1 cup shredded cheddar cheese
- 2 teaspoons olive oil
- Salt and pepper, to taste

Directions:

1. Preheat oven to 350°F.
2. Heat 1 tsp of olive oil in a saucepan over medium-high heat. Sauté garlic for 1 minute until flavored.
3. Add the zucchini and cook for another 5-7 minutes until soft.
4. Beat the eggs and then add a little milk and Parmesan cheese.
5. Meanwhile, heat the remaining olive oil in another saucepan and add the kale. Cover and cook for 5 minutes until dry.
6. Slightly grease a baking dish with cooking spray and spread the kale leaves across the bottom. Add the zucchini and top with goat cheese.
7. Pour the egg, milk, and parmesan mixture evenly over the other ingredients. Top with cheddar cheese.
8. Bake for 50–60 minutes until golden brown. Check the center of the quiche, it should have a solid consistency.
9. Let chill for a few minutes before serving.

Nutrition:

Total Carbohydrates: 15g
Dietary Fiber: 2 g
Net Carbs: 13 g
Protein: 19 g
Total Fat: 18 g
Calories: 290

42. Cream Cheese Egg Breakfast

Preparation Time: 5 minutes

Cooking Time: 5 minutes

Servings: 4

Ingredients:

- 2 eggs, beaten
- 1 tablespoon butter
- 2 tablespoons soft cream cheese with chives

Directions:

1. Melt the butter in a small skillet.
2. Add the eggs and cream cheese.
3. Stir and cook to desired doneness.

Nutrition:

Calories: 341 Fat: 31 g

Protein: 15 g Carbohydrate: 0 g Dietary Fiber: 3 g

43. Avocado Red Peppers Roasted Scrambled Eggs

Preparation Time: 10 minutes

Cooking Time: 12 minutes

Servings: 3

Ingredients:

- 1/2 tablespoon butter
- Eggs, 2
- 1/2 roasted red pepper, about 1 1/2 ounces
- 1/2 small avocado, coarsely chopped, about 2 1/4 ounces
- Salt, to taste

Directions:

1. In a nonstick skillet, heat the butter over medium heat. Break the eggs into the pan and break the yolks with a spoon. Sprinkle with a little salt.
2. Stir to stir and continue stirring until the eggs start to come out. Quickly add the bell peppers and avocado.
3. Cook and stir until the eggs suit your taste. Adjust the seasoning, if necessary.

Nutrition:

Calories: 317 Fat: 26g Protein: 14g

Dietary Fiber: 5g Net Carbs: 4g

44. Mushroom Quickie Scramble

Preparation Time: 10 minutes

Cooking Time: 10 minutes

Servings: 4

Ingredients:

- 3 small-sized eggs, whisked
- 4 pcs. Bella mushrooms
- ½ cup of spinach
- ¼ cup of red bell peppers
- 2 deli ham slices
- 1 tablespoon of ghee or coconut oil
- Salt and pepper to taste

Directions:

1. Chop the ham and veggies.
2. Put half a tbsp. of butter in a frying pan and heat until melted.
3. Sauté the ham and vegetables in a frying pan then set aside.
4. Get a new frying pan and heat the remaining butter.
5. Add the whisked eggs into the second pan while stirring continuously to avoid overcooking.
6. When the eggs are done, sprinkle with salt and pepper to taste.
7. Add the ham and veggies to the pan with the eggs.
8. Mix well.
9. Remove from burner and transfer to a plate.

Nutrition:

Calories: 350 Total Fat: 29 g Protein: 21 g Total Carbs: 5 g

45. Coconut Coffee and Ghee

Preparation Time: 10 minutes

Cooking Time: 10 minutes

Servings: 5

Ingredients:

- ½ Tbsp. of coconut oil
- ½ Tbsp. of ghee
- 1 to 2 cups of preferred coffee (or rooibos or black tea, if preferred)
- 1 Tbsp. of coconut or almond milk

Directions:

1. Place the almond (or coconut) milk, coconut oil, ghee, and coffee in a blender (or milk frother).
2. Mix for around 10 seconds or until the coffee turns creamy and foamy.
3. Pour contents into a coffee cup. Serve immediately and enjoy.

Nutrition:

Calories: 150 Total Fat: 15 g Protein: 0 g Total Carbs: 0 g Net Carbs: 0 g

46. Yummy Veggie Waffles

Preparation Time: 10 minutes

Cooking Time: 9 minutes

Servings: 3

Ingredients:

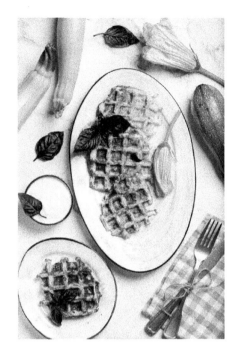

- 3 cups raw cauliflower, grated
- 1 cup cheddar cheese
- 1 cup mozzarella cheese
- ½ cup parmesan
- 1/3 cup chives, finely sliced
- 6 eggs
- 1 teaspoon garlic powder
- 1 teaspoon onion powder
- ½ teaspoon chili flakes
- Dash of salt and pepper

Directions:

1. Turn waffle maker on.
2. In a bowl, mix all the listed ingredients very well until incorporated.
3. Once the waffle maker is hot, distribute the waffle mixture into the insert.
4. Let cook for about 9 minutes, flipping at 6 minutes.
5. Remove from waffle maker and set aside.
6. Serve and enjoy!

Nutrition:

Calories: 390

Fat: 28 g

Carbs: 6 g

Fiber: 2 g

Protein: 30 g

47. Omega 3 Breakfast Shake

Preparation Time: 5 minutes

Cooking Time: 5 minutes

Servings: 2

Ingredients:

- 1 cup vanilla almond milk (unsweetened)
- 2 tablespoons blueberries
- 1 ½ tablespoons flaxseed meal
- 1 tablespoon MCT Oil
- ¾ tablespoon banana extract
- ½ tablespoon chia seeds
- 5 drops Stevia (liquid form)
- 1/8 tablespoon Xanthan gum

Directions:

1. In a blender, mix vanilla almond milk, banana extract, Stevia, and three ice cubes.
2. When smooth, add blueberries and pulse.
3. Once blueberries are thoroughly incorporated, add flaxseed meal and chia seeds.
4. Let sit for 5 minutes.
5. After 5 minutes, pulse again until all ingredients are nicely distributed. Serve and enjoy

Nutrition:

Calories: 264

Fats: 25 g

Carbs: 7 g

Protein: 4 g

CHAPTER 10:

Dinner

48. Brown Basmati Rice Pilaf

Preparation Time: 10 minutes
Cooking Time: 3 minutes
Servings: 2
Ingredients:

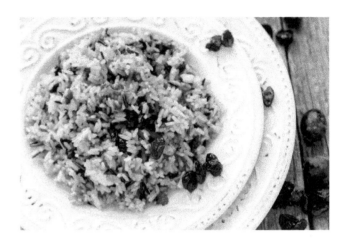

- ½ tablespoon vegan butter
- ½ cup mushrooms, chopped
- ½ cup brown basmati rice
- 2-3 tablespoons water
- 1/8 teaspoon dried thyme
- Ground pepper to taste
- ½ tablespoon olive oil
- ¼ cup green onion, chopped
- 1 cup vegetable broth
- ¼ teaspoon salt
- ¼ cup chopped, toasted pecans

Directions:

1. Place a saucepan over medium-low heat. Add butter and oil.
2. When it melts, add mushrooms and cook until slightly tender.
3. Stir in the green onion and brown rice. Cook for 3 minutes. Stir constantly.
4. Stir in the broth, water, salt, and thyme.
5. When it begins to boil, lower the heat and cover with a lid. Simmer until rice is cooked. Add more water or broth if required.
6. Stir in the pecans and pepper.
7. Serve.

Nutrition:

Calories 189

Fats 11 g

Carbohydrates 19 g

Proteins 4 g

49. Shakshuka

Preparation Time: 10 minutes
Cooking Time: 30 minutes
Servings: 1
Ingredients:

- Chopped parsley, 1 tablespoon
- Extra virgin olive oil, 1 teaspoon
- Paprika, 1 teaspoon
- Red onion, ½ cup (finely chopped)
- Kale, 30g (stems removed and roughly chopped)
- Garlic clove, 1 (finely chopped)
- Celery, 30g (finely chopped)
- Bird's eye chili, 1 (finely chopped)
- Ground turmeric, 1 teaspoon
- Ground cumin, 1 teaspoon
- Tinned chopped tomatoes, 2 cups
- Medium eggs, 2

Directions:

1. Place a small, deep-sided frying pan over medium-low heat. Add the oil once hot, then add the chili, spices, celery, garlic, and onions. Fry for about 2 minutes.
2. Add the tomatoes, then allow the sauce to simmer gently for approx. 20 min while stirring frequently.
3. Add the kale to the pot and cook for another five minutes. Add a little water if the sauce gets too thick. Stir in the parsley once the sauce becomes nicely creamy.
4. Create two little wells in the sauce, then break each egg into the wells. Reduce your heat to the lowest and cover the pan with a foil or with its lid.
5. Allow the eggs to cook for about 10 minutes, or until the whites are firm and the yolks remain runny. Cook for another four minutes if you want the yolks to be firm.
6. Serve immediately.

Nutrition:

Calories: 657

Protein: 87 g

Fat: 4 g

Sugar: 6 g

50. Walnut and Date Porridge

Preparation Time: 10 minutes

Cooking Time: 0 minutes

Servings: 1

Ingredients:

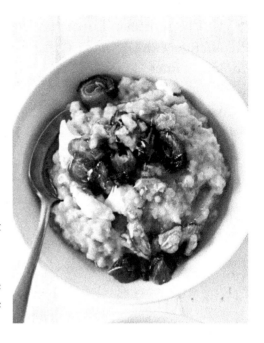

- Strawberries, ½ cup (hulled)
- Milk or dairy-free alternative, 200 ml
- Buckwheat flakes, ½ cup
- Medjool date, 1 (chopped)
- Walnut butter, 1 teaspoon, or chopped walnut halves

Directions:

1. Place the date and the milk in a pan, heat gently before adding the buckwheat flakes. Then cook until the porridge gets to your desired consistency.
2. Add the walnuts, stir, then top with the strawberries.
3. Serve.

Nutrition:

Calories: 254

Protein: 65 g

Fat: 4 g

Vitamin B

51. Vietnamese Turmeric Fish with Mango and Herbs Sauce

Preparation Time: 15 minutes

Cooking Time: 30 minutes

Servings: 4

Ingredients:

For the Fish:

- Coconut oil to fry the fish, 2 tablespoons
- Fresh codfish, skinless and boneless, 1 ¼ lbs. (cut into 2-inch piece wide)
- Pinch of sea salt, to taste

Fish Marinade:

- Chinese cooking wine, 1 tablespoon
- Turmeric powder, 1 tablespoon
- Sea salt, 1 teaspoon
- Olive oil, 2 tablespoons - Minced ginger, 2 teaspoons

Mango Dipping Sauce:

- Juice of ½ lime - Medium-sized ripe mango, 1
- Rice vinegar, 2 tablespoons
- Dry red chili pepper, 1 teaspoon (stir in before serving)
- Garlic clove, 1 - Infused scallion and dill oil
- Fresh dill, 2 cups - Scallions, 2 cups (slice into long thin shape)
- A pinch of sea salt, to taste.

Toppings

- Nuts (pine or cashew nuts) - Lime juice (as much as you like)
- Fresh cilantro (as much as you like)

Directions:

1. Add all the ingredients under "Mango Dipping Sauce" into your food processor. Blend until you get your preferred consistency. Add two tablespoons of coconut oil in a large non-stick frying pan and heat over high heat. Once hot, add the pre-marinated fish. Add the slices of the fish into the pan individually. Divide into batches for easy frying, if necessary. Once you hear a loud sizzle, reduce the heat to medium-high.

2. Do not move or turn the fish until it turns golden brown on one side; then turn it to the other side to fry, about 5 minutes on each side. Add more coconut oil to the pan if needed. Season with the sea salt. Transfer the fish to a large plate. You will have some oil left in the frypan, which you will use to make your scallion and dill infused oil.

3. Using the remaining oil in the frypan, set to medium-high heat, add 2 cups of dill, and 2 cups of scallions. Put off the heat after you have added the dill and scallions. Toss them gently for about 15 seconds, until the dill and scallions have wilted. Add a dash of sea salt to season. Pour the dill, scallion, and infused oil over the fish. Serve with mango dipping sauce, nuts, lime, and fresh cilantro.

Nutrition:

Calories: 234 Fat: 23 g Protein: 76 g Sugar: 5 g

52. Chicken and Kale Curry

Preparation Time: 20 min

Cooking Time: 1 hour

Servings: 3

Ingredients:

- Boiling water, 250 ml
- Skinless and boneless chicken thighs, 7 oz.
- Ground turmeric, 2 tablespoons
- Olive oil, 1 tablespoon
- Red onions, 1 (diced)
- Bird's eye chili, 1 (finely chopped)
- Freshly chopped ginger, ½ tablespoon
- Curry powder, ½ tablespoon
- Garlic, 1 ½ cloves (crushed)
- Cardamom pods, 1
- Tinned coconut milk, light, 100 ml
- Chicken stock, 2 cups
- Tinned chopped tomatoes, 1 cup

Direction:

1. Place the chicken thighs in a non-metallic bowl, add one tablespoon of turmeric and one teaspoon of olive oil. Mix together and keep aside to marinate for approx. 30 minutes.
2. Fry the chicken thighs over medium heat for about 5 minutes until well cooked and brown on all sides. Remove from the pan and set aside.
3. Add the remaining oil into a frypan on medium heat. Then add the onion, ginger, garlic, and chili. Fry for about 10 minutes until soft.
4. Add one tablespoon of the turmeric and half a tablespoon of curry powder to the pan and cook for another 2 minutes.
5. Then add the cardamom pods, coconut milk, tomatoes, and chicken stock. Allow simmering for thirty minutes.
6. Add the chicken once the sauce has reduced a little into the pan, followed by the kale. Cook until the kale is tender and the chicken is warm enough.
7. Serve with buckwheat.
8. Garnish with the chopped coriander.

Nutrition:

Calories: 313 g

Protein: 13 g

Fat: 6 g

Carbohydrate: 23 g

53. Mediterranean Baked Penne

Preparation Time: 25 minutes
Cooking Time: 1 hour 20 minutes
Servings: 8
Ingredients:

- Extra-virgin olive oil, 1 tablespoon
- Fine dry breadcrumbs, ½ cup
- Small zucchini, 2 (chopped)
- Medium eggplant, 1 (chopped)
- Medium onion, 1 (chopped)
- Red bell pepper, 1 (seeded and chopped)
- Celery, 1 stalk (sliced)
- Garlic, 1 clove (minced)
- Salt and freshly ground pepper to taste
- Dry white wine, ¼ cup
- Plum tomatoes, 28-ounces (drained and coarsely chopped, juice reserved)
- Freshly grated Parmesan cheese, 2 tablespoons
- Large eggs, 2 (lightly beaten)
- Coarsely grated part-skim mozzarella cheese, 1 ½ cups
- Dried penne rig ate or rigatoni, 1 pound

Directions:

1. Preheat your oven to 375 degrees F. Apply nonstick spray on a 3-quart baking dish. Then coat the dish with ¼ cup of breadcrumbs, tapping out the excess.
2. Heat the oil in a large non-stick skillet over medium-high heat. Then add the onion, celery, bell pepper, eggplant, and zucchini.
3. Cook for about 10 minutes, occasionally stirring, until smooth. Then add the garlic and cook for another minute. Add the wine, stir and cook for about 2 minutes, long enough for the wine to almost evaporate.
4. Then add the juice and tomatoes. Bring to a simmer, then cook for about 10 to 15 minutes, until thickened, season with pepper and salt.
5. Transfer to a large bowl and allow to cool.
6. Pour water into a pot, add some salt, and then allow to boil. Add the penne into the boiling salted water to cook for about 10 minutes, until al dente.
7. Drain and rinse the pasta under running water. Toss the pasta with the vegetable mixture, then stir in the mozzarella.
8. Scoop the pasta mixture and place into the prepared baking dish. Drizzle the broken eggs evenly over the top.
9. Mix the Parmesan and ¼ cups of breadcrumbs in a small bowl, then sprinkle evenly over the top of the dish. Place the dish into the oven to bake for about 40 to 50 minutes, until bubbly and golden.
10. Allow to rest for 10 min before you serve.

Nutrition:
Calories: 372 Protein: 45 g Fat: 8 g Sugar: 2 g

54. Prawn Arrabbiata

Preparation Time: 35 minutes

Cooking Time: 30 minutes

Servings: 1

Ingredients:

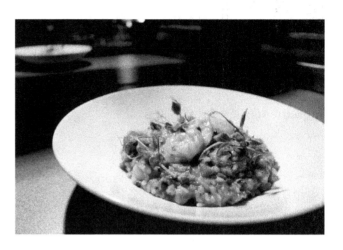

- Raw or cooked prawns, 1 cup
- Extra virgin olive oil, 1 tablespoon
- Buckwheat pasta, ½ cup
- Chopped parsley, 1 tablespoon
- Celery, ¼ cup (finely chopped)
- Tinned chopped tomatoes, 2 cups
- Red onion, 1/3 cup (finely chopped)
- Garlic clove, 1 (finely chopped)
- Extra virgin olive oil, 1 teaspoon
- Dried mixed herbs, 1 teaspoon
- Bird's eye chili, 1 (finely chopped)
- White wine, 2 tablespoons (optional)

Directions:

1. Add the olive oil into your fry-pan and fry the dried herbs, celery, and onions over medium-low heat for about two minutes.
2. Increase heat to medium, add the wine and cook for another min.
3. Add the tomatoes to the pan and allow to simmer for about 30 minutes, over medium-low heat, until you get a nice creamy consistency.
4. Add a little water if the sauce gets too thick.
5. While the sauce is cooking, cook the pasta following the instruction on the packet. Drain the water once the pasta is done cooking, toss with the olive oil, and set aside until needed.
6. If using raw prawns, add them to your sauce and cook for another four minutes, until the prawns turn opaque and pink, then add the parsley. If using cooked prawns, add them at the same time with the parsley and allow the sauce to boil.
7. Add the already cooked pasta to the sauce, mix them, and serve.

Nutrition:

Calories: 321

Protein: 19 g

Fat: 2 g

Carbohydrate: 23 g

55. Barb's Asian Slaw

Preparation Time: 5 minutes
Cooking Time: 5 minutes
Servings: 2
Ingredients:

- 1 cabbage head, shredded
- 4 chopped green onions
- ½ cup slivered or sliced almonds

Dressing:

- ½ cup olive oil
- ¼ cup tamari or soy sauce
- 1 tablespoon honey or maple syrup
- 1 tablespoon baking stevia

Directions:

1. Heat up dressing ingredients in a saucepan on the stove until thoroughly mixed.
2. Mix all ingredients when you are ready to serve.

Nutrition:

Calories: 205

Protein: 27g

Carbohydrate: 12g

Fat: 10 g

56. Blueberry Cantaloupe Avocado Salad

Preparation Time: 5 minutes
Cooking Time: 0 minutes
Servings: 2
Ingredients:

- 1 diced cantaloupe
- 2–3 chopped avocados
- 1 package of blueberries
- ¼ cup olive oil
- 1/8 cup balsamic vinegar

Directions:

1. Mix all ingredients.

Nutrition:

Calories: 406

Protein: 9g

Carbohydrate: 32g

Fat: 5 g

57. Beet Salad (from Israel)

Preparation Time: 5 minutes

Cooking Time: 0 minutes

Servings: 2

Ingredients:

- 2–3 fresh, raw beets grated or shredded in food processor
- 3 tablespoons olive oil
- 2 tablespoons balsamic vinegar
- ¼ teaspoon salt
- 1/3 teaspoon cumin
- Dash stevia powder or liquid
- Dash pepper

Directions:

1. Mix all ingredients together for the best raw beet salad.

Nutrition:

Calories: 156

Protein: 8g

Carbohydrate: 40g

Fat: 5 g

58. Broccoli Salad

Preparation Time: 5 minutes

Cooking Time: 0 minutes

Servings: 2

Ingredients:

- 1 head broccoli, chopped
- 2–3 slices of fried bacon, crumbled
- 1 diced green onion
- ½ cup raisins or craisins
- ½–1 cup of chopped pecans
- ¾ cup sunflower seeds
- ½ cup of pomegranate

Dressing:

- 1 cup organic mayonnaise
- ¼ cup baking stevia
- 2 teaspoons white vinegar

Directions:

1. Mix all ingredients together. Mix dressing and fold into salad.

Nutrition:

Calories: 239 Protein: 10g Carbohydrate: 33g Fat: 2 g

59. Rosemary Garlic Potatoes

Preparation Time: 5 minutes

Cooking Time: 30 minutes

Servings: 2

Ingredients:

- 5 red new potatoes, chopped
- ¼ cup olive oil
- 2–3 cloves of minced garlic
- 1 tablespoon rosemary

Directions:

1. Preheat oven to 425 degrees.
2. Stir all ingredients together in a bowl. Pour onto a baking sheet and bake for 30 minutes.

Nutrition:

Calories: 176

Protein: 5g

Carbohydrate: 30g

Fat: 2 g

60. Sweet and Sour Cabbage

Preparation Time: 5 minutes

Cooking Time: 15 minutes

Servings: 2

Ingredients:

- 1 tablespoon honey or maple syrup
- 1 teaspoon baking stevia
- 2 tablespoons water
- 1 tablespoon olive oil
- ¼ teaspoon caraway seeds
- ¼ teaspoon salt
- 1/8 teaspoon pepper
- 2 cups chopped red cabbage
- 1 diced apple

Directions:

1. Cook all ingredients in a covered saucepan on the stove for 15 minutes.

Nutrition:

Calories: 170

Protein: 17g

Carbohydrate: 20g

Fat: 8 g

61. Barley and Lentil Salad

Preparation Time: 5 minutes

Cooking Time: 0 minutes

Servings: 2

Ingredients:

- 1 head romaine lettuce
- ¾ cup cooked barley
- 2 cups cooked lentils
- 1 diced carrot
- ¼ chopped red onion
- ¼ cup olives
- ½ chopped cucumber
- 3 tablespoons olive oil
- 2 tablespoons fresh lemon juice

Directions:

1. Mix all ingredients together. Add kosher salt and black pepper to taste.

Nutrition:

Calories: 213

Protein: 21g

Carbohydrate: 6g

Fat: 9 g

62. Taste of Normandy Salad

Preparation Time: 25 minutes

Cooking Time: 5 minutes

Servings: 4 to 6

Ingredients:

For the walnuts:

- 2 tablespoons butter
- ¼ cup sugar or honey
- 1 cup walnut pieces
- ½ teaspoon kosher salt
- For the dressing
- 3 tablespoons extra-virgin olive oil
- 1½ tablespoons champagne vinegar
- 1½ tablespoons Dijon mustard
- ¼ teaspoon kosher salt

For the salad:

- 1 head red leaf lettuce, torn into pieces
- 3 heads endive, ends trimmed and leaves separated
- 2 apples, cored and cut into thin wedges
- 1 (8-ounce) Camembert wheel, cut into thin wedges

Directions:

2. To make the walnuts
3. In a skillet over medium-high heat, melt the butter. Stir in the sugar and cook until it dissolves. Add the walnuts and cook for about 5 minutes, stirring, until toasty. Season with salt and transfer to a plate to cool.
4. To make the dressing
5. In a large bowl, whisk the oil, vinegar, mustard, and salt until combined.
6. To make the salad
7. Add the lettuce and endive to the bowl with the dressing and toss to coat. Transfer to a serving platter.
8. Decoratively arrange the apple and Camembert wedges over the lettuce and scatter the walnuts on top. Serve immediately.

Nutrition:

Calories: 699;

Total fat: 52g;

Total carbs: 44g;

Cholesterol: 60mg;

Fiber: 17g;

Protein: 23g;

Sodium: 1170mg

63. Norwegian Niçoise Salad: Smoked Salmon, Cucumber, Egg, and Asparagus

Preparation Time: 20 minutes

Cooking Time: 5 minutes

Servings: 4

Ingredients:

- For the vinaigrette
- 3 tablespoons walnut oil
- 2 tablespoons champagne vinegar
- 1 tablespoon chopped fresh dill
- ½ teaspoon kosher salt
- ¼ teaspoon ground mustard
- Freshly ground black pepper

For the salad:

- Handful green beans, trimmed
- 1 (3- to 4-ounce) package spring greens
- 12 spears pickled asparagus
- 4 large soft-boiled eggs, halved
- 8 ounces smoked salmon, thinly sliced
- 1 cucumber, thinly sliced
- 1 lemon, quartered

Directions:

1. To make the dressing
2. In a small bowl, whisk the oil, vinegar, dill, salt, ground mustard, and a few grinds of pepper until emulsified. Set aside.
3. To make the salad
4. Start by blanching the green beans: Bring a pot of salted water to a boil. Drop in the beans. Cook or 1 to 2 minutes until they turn bright green, then immediately drain and rinse under cold water. Set aside.
5. Divide the spring greens among 4 plates. Toss each serving with dressing to taste. Arrange 3 asparagus spears, 1 egg, 2 ounces of salmon, one-fourth of the cucumber slices, and a lemon wedge on each plate. Serve immediately.

Nutrition:

Calories: 257;

Total fat: 18g;

Total carbs: 6g;

Cholesterol: 199mg;

Fiber: 2g;

Protein: 19g;

Sodium: 603mg

CHAPTER 11:

Dinner Recipes

64. Warm Chorizo Chickpea Salad

Preparation Time: 5 minutes
Cooking Time: 20 minutes
Servings: 6
Ingredients:

- 1 tablespoon extra-virgin olive oil
- 4 chorizo links, sliced
- 1 red onion, sliced
- 4 roasted red bell peppers, chopped
- 1 can chickpeas, drained
- 2 cups cherry tomatoes
- 2 tablespoons balsamic vinegar
- Salt and pepper to taste

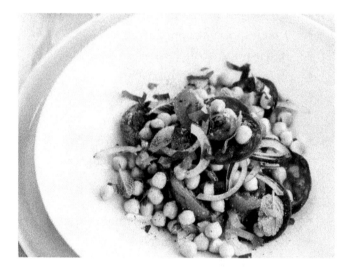

Directions:

1. Heat the oil in a skillet and add the chorizo. Cook briefly just until fragrant then add the onion, bell peppers and chickpeas and cook for 2 additional minutes.
2. Transfer the mixture in a salad bowl then add the tomatoes, vinegar, salt and pepper.
3. Mix well and serve the salad right away.

Nutrition:

Calories: 359

Fat: 18g

Protein: 15g

Carbohydrates: 21g

65. Greek Roasted Fish

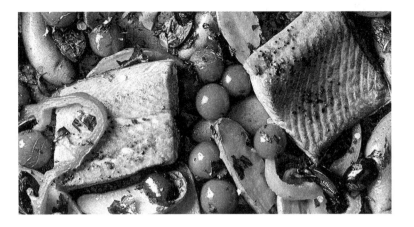

Preparation Time: 5 minutes
Cooking Time: 30 minutes
Servings: 4
Ingredients:

- 4 salmon fillets
- 1 tablespoon chopped oregano
- 1 teaspoon dried basil
- 1 zucchini, sliced
- 1 red onion, sliced
- 1 carrot, sliced
- 1 lemon, sliced
- 2 tablespoons extra virgin olive oil
- Salt and pepper to taste

Directions:

1. Add all the ingredients in a deep dish baking pan.
2. Season with salt and pepper and cook in the preheated oven at 350F for 20 minutes.
3. Serve the fish and vegetables warm.

Nutrition:

Calories: 328

Fat: 13g

Protein: 38g

Carbohydrates: 8g

66. Tomato Fish Bake

Preparation Time: 5 minutes
Cooking Time: 30 minutes
Servings: 4
Ingredients:

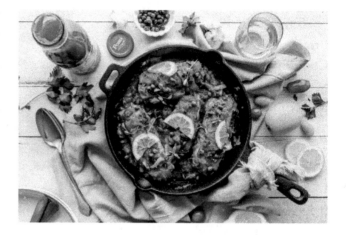

- 4 cod fillets
- 4 tomatoes, sliced
- 4 garlic cloves, minced
- 1 shallot, sliced
- 1 celery stalk, sliced
- 1 teaspoon fennel seeds
- 1 cup vegetable stock
- Salt and pepper to taste

Directions:

1. Layer the cod fillets and tomatoes in a deep dish baking pan.
2. Add the rest of the ingredients and add salt and pepper.
3. Cook in the preheated oven at 350F for 20 minutes.
4. Serve the dish warm or chilled.

Nutrition:

Calories: 299

Fat: 3g

Protein: 64g

Carbohydrates: 2g

67. Garlicky Tomato Chicken Casserole

Preparation Time: 5 minutes

Cooking Time: 50 minutes

Servings: 4

Ingredients:

- 4 chicken breasts
- 2 tomatoes, sliced
- 1 can diced tomatoes
- 2 garlic cloves, chopped
- 1 shallot, chopped
- 1 bay leaf
- 1 thyme sprig
- ½ cup dry white wine
- ½ cup chicken stock
- Salt and pepper to taste

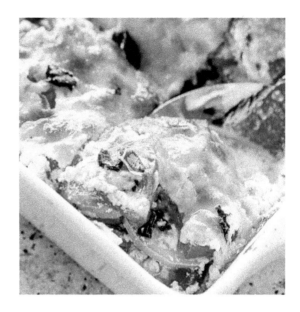

Directions:

1. Combine the chicken and the remaining ingredients in a deep dish baking pan.
2. Adjust the taste with salt and pepper and cover the pot with a lid or aluminum foil.
3. Cook in the preheated oven at 330F for 40 minutes.
4. Serve the casserole warm.

Nutrition:

Calories: 313

Fat: 8g

Protein: 47g

Carbohydrates: 6g

68. Chicken Cacciatore

Preparation Time: 5 minutes
Cooking Time: 45 minutes
Servings: 6
Ingredients:

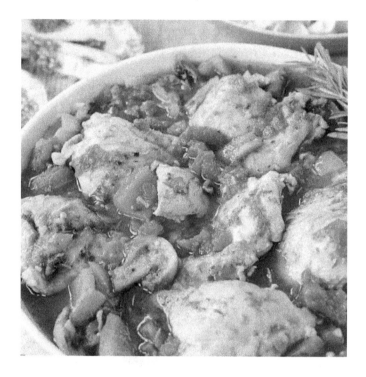

- 2 tablespoons extra virgin olive oil
- 6 chicken thighs
- 1 sweet onion, chopped
- 2 garlic cloves, minced
- 2 red bell peppers, cored and diced
- 2 carrots, diced
- 1 rosemary sprig
- 1 thyme sprig
- 4 tomatoes, peeled and diced
- ½ cup tomato juice
- ¼ cup dry white wine
- 1 cup chicken stock
- 1 bay leaf
- Salt and pepper to taste

Directions:

1. Heat the oil in a heavy saucepan.
2. Cook chicken on all sides until golden.
3. Stir in the onion and garlic and cook for 2 minutes.
4. Stir in the rest of the ingredients and season with salt and pepper.
5. Cook on low heat for 30 minutes.
6. Serve the chicken cacciatore warm and fresh.

Nutrition:

Calories: 363

Fat: 14g

Protein: 42g

Carbohydrates: 9g

69. Fennel Wild Rice Risotto

Preparation Time: 5 minutes

Cooking Time: 35 minutes

Servings: 6

Ingredients:

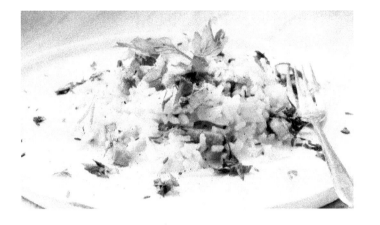

- 2 tablespoons extra virgin olive oil
- 1 shallot, chopped
- 2 garlic cloves, minced
- 1 fennel bulb, chopped
- 1 cup wild rice
- ¼ cup dry white wine
- 2 cups chicken stock
- 1 teaspoon grated orange zest
- Salt and pepper to taste

Directions:

1. Heat the oil in a heavy saucepan.
2. Add the garlic, shallot and fennel and cook for a few minutes until softened.
3. Stir in the rice and cook for 2 additional minutes then add the wine, stock and orange zest, with salt and pepper to taste.
4. Cook on low heat for 20 minutes.
5. Serve the risotto warm and fresh.

Nutrition:

Calories: 162

Fat: 2g

Protein: 8g

Carbohydrates: 20g

70. Wild Rice Prawn Salad

Preparation Time: 5 minutes

Cooking Time: 35 minutes

Servings: 6

Ingredients:

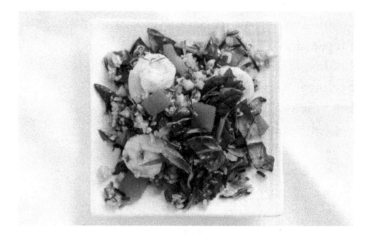

- ¾ cup wild rice
- 1¾ cups chicken stock
- 1 pound prawns
- Salt and pepper to taste
- 2 tablespoons lemon juice
- 2 tablespoons extra virgin olive oil
- 2 cups arugula

Directions:

1. Combine the rice and chicken stock in a saucepan and cook until the liquid has been absorbed entirely.
2. Transfer the rice in a salad bowl.
3. Season the prawns with salt and pepper and drizzle them with lemon juice and oil.
4. Heat a grill pan over medium flame.
5. Place the prawns on the hot pan and cook on each side for 2-3 minutes.
6. For the salad, combine the rice with arugula and prawns and mix well.
7. Serve the salad fresh.

Nutrition:

Calories: 207

Fat: 4g

Protein: 20.6g

Carbohydrates: 17g

71. Chicken Broccoli Salad with Avocado Dressing

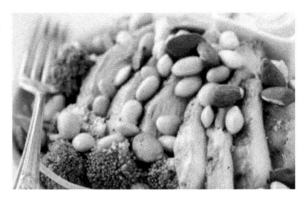

Preparation Time: 5 minutes

Cooking Time: 40 minutes

Servings: 6

Ingredients:

- 2 chicken breasts
- 1 pound broccoli, cut into florets
- 1 avocado, peeled and pitted
- ½ lemon, juiced
- 2 garlic cloves
- ¼ teaspoon chili powder
- ¼ teaspoon cumin powder
- Salt and pepper to taste

Directions:

1. Cook the chicken in a large pot of salty water.
2. Drain and cut the chicken into small cubes. Place in a salad bowl.
3. Add the broccoli and mix well.
4. Combine the avocado, lemon juice, garlic, chili powder, cumin powder, salt and pepper in a blender. Pulse until smooth.
5. Spoon the dressing over the salad and mix well.
6. Serve the salad fresh.

Nutrition:

Calories: 195

Fat: 11g

Protein: 14g

Carbohydrates: 3g

72. Seafood Paella

Preparation Time: 5 minutes

Cooking Time: 45 minutes

Servings: 8

Ingredients:

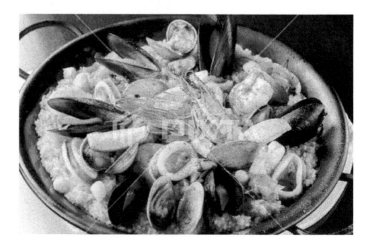

- 2 tablespoons extra virgin olive oil
- 1 shallot, chopped
- 2 garlic cloves, chopped
- 1 red bell pepper, cored and diced
- 1 carrot, diced
- 2 tomatoes, peeled and diced
- 1 cup wild rice
- 1 cup tomato juice
- 2 cups chicken stock
- 1 chicken breast, cubed
- Salt and pepper to taste
- 2 monkfish fillets, cubed
- ½ pound fresh shrimps, peeled and deveined
- ½ pound prawns
- 1 thyme sprig
- 1 rosemary sprig

Directions:

1. Heat the oil in a skillet and stir in the shallot, garlic, bell pepper, carrot and tomatoes. Cook for a few minutes until softened.
2. Stir in the rice, tomato juice, stock, chicken, salt and pepper and cook on low heat for 20 minutes.
3. Add the rest of the ingredients and cook for 10 additional minutes.
4. Serve the paella warm and fresh.

Nutrition:

Calories: 245

Fat: 8g

Protein: 27g

Carbohydrates: 20.6g

73. Herbed Roasted Chicken Breasts

Preparation Time: 5 minutes

Cooking Time: 50 minutes

Servings: 4

Ingredients:

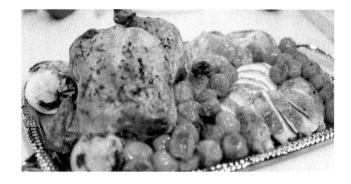

- 2 tablespoons extra virgin olive oil
- 2 tablespoons chopped parsley
- 2 tablespoons chopped cilantro
- 1 teaspoon dried oregano
- 1 teaspoon dried basil
- 2 tablespoons lemon juice
- Salt and pepper to taste
- 4 chicken breasts

Directions:

1. Combine the oil, parsley, cilantro, oregano, basil, lemon juice, salt and pepper in a bowl.
2. Spread this mixture over the chicken and rub it well into the meat.
3. Place in a deep dish baking pan and cover with aluminum foil.
4. Cook in the preheated oven at 350F for 20 minutes then remove the foil and cook for 25 additional minutes.
5. Serve the chicken warm and fresh with your favorite side dish.

Nutrition:

Calories: 330

Fat: 15g

Protein: 40.7g

Carbohydrates: 1g

74. Marinated Chicken Breasts

Preparation Time: 5 minutes
Cooking Time: 2 hours
Servings: 4
Ingredients:

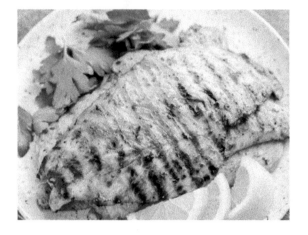

- 4 chicken breasts
- Salt and pepper to taste
- 1 lemon, juiced
- 1 rosemary sprig
- 1 thyme sprig
- 2 garlic cloves, crushed
- 2 sage leaves
- 3 tablespoons extra virgin olive oil
- ½ cup buttermilk

Directions:

1. 1. Boil the chicken with salt and pepper and place it in a resealable bag.
2. 2. Add remaining ingredients and seal bag.
3. 3. Refrigerate for at least 1 hour.
4. 4. After 1 hour, heat a roasting pan over medium heat, then place the chicken on the grill.
5. 5. Cook on each side for 8-10 minutes or until juices are gone.
6. Serve the chicken warm with your favorite side dish.

Nutrition:

Calories: 371

Fat: 21g

Protein: 46g

Carbohydrates: 2g

CHAPTER 12:

Desserts

75. Yogurt Mint

Preparation Time: 5 minutes
Cooking Time: 10 minutes
Servings: 2
Ingredients:

- 1 cup of water
- 5 cups of milk
- ¾ cup plain yogurt
- ¼ cup fresh mint
- 1 tbsp. maple syrup

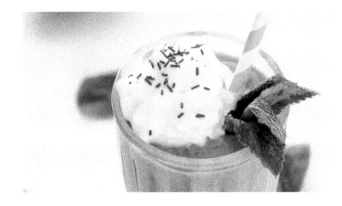

Directions:

1. Add 1 cup water to the Instant Pot Pressure Cooker.
2. Press the STEAM function button and adjust to 1 minute.
3. Once done, add the milk, then press the YOGURT function button and allow boiling.
4. Add yogurt and fresh mint, then stir well.
5. Pour into a glass and add maple syrup.
6. Enjoy.

Nutrition:

Calories: 25

Fat: 0.5 g

Carbs: 5 g

Protein: 2 g

76. Chocolate Fondue

Preparation Time: 5 minutes
Cooking Time: 10 minutes
Servings: 2
Ingredients:

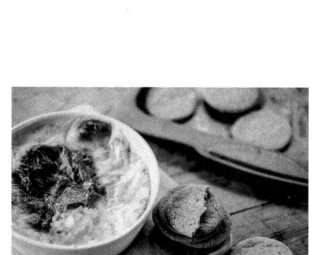

- 1 cup water
- ½ tsp. sugar
- ½ cup coconut cream
- ¾ cup dark chocolate, chopped

Directions:

1. Pour the water into your Instant Pot.
2. To a heatproof bowl, add the chocolate, sugar, and coconut cream.
3. Place in the Instant Pot.
4. Seal the lid, select MANUAL, and cook for 2 minutes. When ready, do a quick release and carefully open the lid. Stir well and serve immediately.

Nutrition:

Calories: 216

Fat: 17 g

Carbs: 11 g

Protein: 2 g

77. Rice Pudding

Preparation Time: 5 minutes
Cooking Time: 12 minutes
Servings: 2
Ingredients:

- ½ cup short grain rice
- ¼ cup of sugar
- 1 cinnamon stick
- 1½ cup milk
- 1 slice lemon peel
- Salt to taste

Directions:

1. Rinse the rice under cold water.
2. Put the milk, cinnamon stick, sugar, salt, and lemon peel inside the Instant Pot Pressure Cooker.
3. Close the lid, lock in place, and make sure to seal the valve. Press the PRESSURE button and cook for 10 minutes on HIGH.
4. When the timer beeps, choose the QUICK PRESSURE release. This will take about 2 minutes.
5. Remove the lid. Open the pressure cooker and discard the lemon peel and cinnamon stick. Spoon in a serving bowl and serve.

Nutrition:

Calories: 111 Fat: 6 g Carbs: 21 g Protein: 3 g

78. Braised Apples

Preparation Time: 5 minutes

Cooking Time: 12 minutes

Servings: 2

Ingredients:

- 2 cored apples
- ½ cup of water
- ½ cup red wine
- 3 tbsp. sugar
- ½ tsp. ground cinnamon

Directions:

1. In the bottom of Instant Pot, add the water and place apples.
2. Pour wine on top and sprinkle with sugar and cinnamon. Close the lid carefully and cook for 10 minutes at HIGH PRESSURE.
3. When done, do a quick pressure release.
4. Transfer the apples onto serving plates and top with cooking liquid.
5. Serve immediately.

Nutrition:

Calories: 245 Fat: 0.5 g Carbs: 53 g Protein: 1 g

79. Wine Figs

Preparation Time: 5 minutes

Cooking Time: 3 minutes

Servings: 2

Ingredients:

- ½ cup pine nuts
- 1 cup red wine
- 1 lb. figs
- Sugar, as needed

Directions:

1. Slowly pour the wine and sugar into the Instant Pot.
2. Arrange the trivet inside it; place the figs over it. Close the lid and lock. Ensure that you have sealed the valve to avoid leakage.
3. Press MANUAL mode and set timer to 3 minutes.
4. After the timer reads zero, press CANCEL and quick-release pressure.
5. Carefully remove the lid.
6. Divide figs into bowls, and drizzle wine from the pot over them.
7. Top with pine nuts and enjoy.

Nutrition:

Calories: 95 Fat: 3 g Carbs: 5 g Protein: 2 g

80. Lemon Curd

Preparation Time: 10 minutes

Cooking Time: 10 minutes

Servings: 2

Ingredients:

- 4 tbsp. butter
- 1 cup sugar
- 2/3 cup lemon juice
- 3 eggs
- 2 tsp. lemon zest
- 1 ½ cups of water

Directions:

1. Whisk the butter and sugar thoroughly until smooth.
2. Add 2 whole eggs and incorporate just the yolk of the other egg.
3. Add the lemon juice.
4. Transfer the mixture into the two jars and tightly seal the tops
5. Pour 1 ½ cups of water into the bottom of the Instant Pot and place in steaming rack. Put the jars on the rack and cook on HIGH PRESSURE for 10 minutes.
6. Natural-release the pressure for 10 minutes before quick releasing the rest.
7. Stir in the zest and put the lids back on the jars.

Nutrition:

Calories: 45

Fat: 1 g

Carbs: 8 g

Protein: 1 g

81. Rhubarb Dessert

Preparation Time: 4 minutes

Cooking Time: 5 minutes

Servings: 2

Ingredients:

- 3 cups rhubarb, chopped
- 1 tbsp. ghee, melted
- 1/3 cup water
- 1 tbsp. stevia
- 1 tsp. vanilla extract

Directions:

1. Put all the listed **Ingredients:** in your Instant Pot, cover, and cook on HIGH for 5 minutes.
2. Divide into small bowls and serve cold.
3. Enjoy!

Nutrition:

Calories: 83 Fat: 2 g Carbs: 2 g Protein: 2 g

82. Raspberry Compote

Preparation Time: 11 minutes

Cooking Time: 30 minutes

Servings: 2

Ingredients:

- 1 cup raspberries
- ½ cup Swerve
- 1 tsp freshly grated lemon zest
- 1 tsp vanilla extract
- 2 cups water

Directions:

1. Press the SAUTÉ button on your Instant Pot, then add all the listed Ingredients.
2. Stir well and pour in 1 cup of water.
3. Cook for 5 minutes, continually stirring, then pour in 1 more cup of water and press the CANCEL button.
4. Secure the lid properly, press the MANUAL button, and set the timer to 15 minutes on LOW pressure.
5. When the timer buzzes, press the CANCEL button and release the pressure naturally for 10minutes.
6. Move the pressure handle to the "venting" position to release any remaining pressure and open the lid.
7. Let it cool before serving.

Nutrition:

Calories: 48 Fat: 0.5 g Carbs: 5 g Protein: 1 g

83. Poached Pears

Preparation Time: 8 minutes

Cooking Time: 10 minutes

Servings: 2

Ingredients:

- 1 tbsp. lime juice
- 2 tsp. lime zest
- 1 cinnamon stick
- 2 whole pears, peeled
- 1 cup of water
- Fresh mint leaves for garnish

Directions:

1. Add all **Ingredients:** except for the mint leaves to the Instant Pot.
2. Seal the Instant Pot and choose the MANUAL button.
3. Cook on HIGH for 10 minutes.
4. Perform a natural pressure release.
5. Remove the pears from the pot. Serve in bowls and garnish with mint on top.

Nutrition:

Calories: 59 Fat: 0.1 g Carbs: 14 g Protein: 0.3 g

84. Apple Crisp

Preparation Time: 10 minutes
Cooking Time: 13 minutes
Servings: 2
Ingredients:

- 2 apples, sliced into chunks
- 1 tsp. cinnamon
- ¼ cup rolled oats
- 1/4 cup brown sugar
- ½ cup of water

Directions:

1. Put all the listed **Ingredients:** in the pot and mix well.
2. Seal the pot, choose MANUAL mode, and cook at HIGH pressure for 8 minutes.
3. Release the pressure naturally and let sit for 5 minutes or until the sauce has thickened.
4. Serve and enjoy.

Nutrition:

Calories: 218

Fat: 5 mg

Carbs: 54 g

CHAPTER 13:

Dessert Recipes

85. Simple Cheesecake

Preparation Time: 10 minutes
Cooking Time: 15 Minutes
Servings: 15
Ingredients:

- 1 lb. cream cheese
- ½ tbsp. vanilla extract
- 2 eggs
- 4 tbsp. sugar
- 1 cup graham crackers
- 2 tbsp. butter

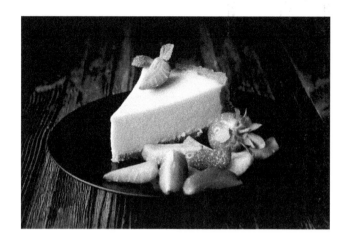

Directions:

1. Mix in butter with crackers in a bowl.
2. Compress crackers blend to the bottom cake pan, put into air fryer and cook at 350° F for 4 minutes.
3. Mix cream cheese with sugar, vanilla, egg in a bowl and beat properly.
4. Sprinkle filling on crackers crust and cook cheesecake in air fryer at 310° F for 15 minutes.
5. Keep cake in fridge for 3 hours, slice.
6. Serve.

Nutrition: Calories: 257

Total Fat: 18g

Total carbs: 22g

86. Bread Pudding

Preparation Time: 10 minutes

Cooking Time: 10 Minutes

Servings: 4

Ingredients:

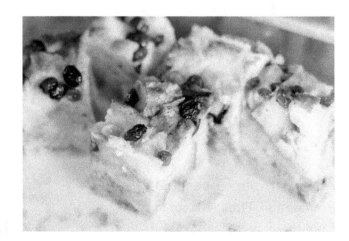

- 6 glazed doughnuts
- 1 cup cherries
- 4 egg yolks
- 1 and ½ cups whipping cream
- ½ cup raisins
- ¼ cup sugar
- ½ cup chocolate chips.

Directions:

1. Mix in cherries with whipping cream and egg in a bowl then turn properly.
2. Mix in raisins with chocolate chips, sugar and doughnuts in a bowl then stir.
3. Mix the 2 mixtures, pour into oiled pan then into air fryer and cook at 310° F for 1 hour.
4. Cool pudding before cutting.
5. Serve.

Nutrition:

Calories: 456 Total Fat: 11g Total carbs: 6g

87. Bread Dough and Amaretto Dessert

Preparation Time: 15 minutes

Cooking Time: 8 Minutes

Servings: 12

Ingredients:

- 1 lb. bread dough
- 1 cup sugar
- ½ cup butter
- 1 cup heavy cream
- 12 oz. chocolate chips
- 2 tbsp. amaretto liqueur

Directions:

1. Turn dough, cut into 20 slices and cut each piece in halves.
2. Sweep dough pieces with spray sugar, butter, put into air fryer's basket and cook them at 350°F for 5 minutes. Turn them, cook for 3 minutes still. Move to a platter.
3. Melt the heavy cream in pan over medium heat, put chocolate chips and turn until they melt.
4. Put in liqueur, turn and move to a bowl.
5. Serve bread dippers with the sauce.

Nutrition:

Calories: 179 Total Fat: 18g Total carbs: 17g

88. Wrapped Pears

Preparation Time: 10 minutes

Cooking Time: 10 Minutes

Servings: 4

Ingredients:

- 4 puff pastry sheets
- 14 oz. vanilla custard
- 2 pears
- 1 egg
- ½ tbsp. cinnamon powder
- 2 tbsp. sugar

Directions:

1. Put wisp pastry slices on flat surface, add spoonful of vanilla custard at the center of each, add pear halves and wrap.
2. Sweep pears with egg, cinnamon and spray sugar, put into air fryer's basket and cook at 320°F for 15 minutes.
3. Split parcels on plates.
4. Serve.

Nutrition:

Calories: 285 Total Fat: 14g Total carbs: 30g

89. Ginger Cheesecake

Preparation Time: 20 minutes

Cooking Time: 20 Minutes

Servings: 6

Ingredients:

- 2 tbsp. butter
- ½ cup ginger cookies
- 16 oz. cream cheese
- 2 eggs
- ½ cup sugar
- 1 tbsp. rum
- ½ tbsp. vanilla extract
- ½ tbsp. nutmeg

Directions:

1. Spread pan with the butter and sprinkle cookie crumbs on the bottom.
2. Whisk cream cheese with rum, vanilla, nutmeg and eggs, beat properly and sprinkle the cookie crumbs.
3. Put in air fryer and cook at 340° F for 20 minutes.
4. Allow cheese cake to cool in fridge for 2 hours before slicing. Serve.

Nutrition:

Calories: 312 Total Fat: 9.8g Total carbs: 18g

90. Cocoa Cookies

Preparation Time: 10 minutes
Cooking Time: 14 Minutes
Servings: 12
Ingredients:

- 6 oz. coconut oil
- 6 eggs
- 3 oz. cocoa powder
- 2 tbsp. vanilla
- ½ tbsp. baking powder
- 4 oz. cream cheese
- 5 tbsp. sugar

Directions:

1. Mix in eggs with coconut oil, baking powder, cocoa powder, cream cheese, vanilla in a blender and sway and turn using a mixer.
2. Get it into a lined baking dish and into the fryer at 320°F and bake for 14 minutes.
3. Split cookie sheet into rectangles.
4. Serve.

Nutrition:
Calories: 149
Total Fat: 2.4g
Total carbs: 27.2g

91. Apple Couscous Pudding

Preparation Time: 10 minutes
Cooking Time: 25 minutes
Servings: 4
Ingredients:

- ½ cup couscous
- 1 and ½ cups milk
- ¼ cup apple, cored and chopped
- 3 tablespoons stevia
- ½ teaspoon rose water
- 1 tablespoon orange zest, grated

Directions:

1. Heat up a pan with the milk over medium heat,
2. Add the couscous and the rest of the ingredients, whisk, simmer for 25 minutes, divide into bowls and serve.

Nutrition:
Calories 150 Fat 4.5 Fiber 5.5
Carbs 7.5 Protein 4

92. Ricotta Ramekins

Preparation Time: 10 minutes

Cooking Time: 1 hour

Servings: 4

Ingredients:

- 6 eggs, whisked
- 1 and ½ pounds ricotta cheese, soft
- ½ pound stevia
- 1 teaspoon vanilla extract
- ½ teaspoon baking powder
- Cooking spray

Directions:

1. In a bowl, mix the eggs with the ricotta and the other ingredients except the cooking spray and whisk well.
2. Grease 4 ramekins with the cooking spray, pour the ricotta cream in each and bake at 360 degrees F for 1 hour.
3. Serve cold.

Nutrition:

Calories 180

Fat 5.3

Fiber 5.4

Carbs 11.5

Protein 4

93. Papaya Cream

Preparation Time: 10 minutes

Cooking Time: 0 minutes

Servings: 2

Ingredients:

- 1 cup papaya, peeled and chopped
- 1 cup heavy cream
- 1 tablespoon stevia
- ½ teaspoon vanilla extract

Directions:

1. In a blender, combine the cream with the papaya and the other ingredients, pulse well, divide into cups and serve cold.

Nutrition:

Calories 182

Fat 3.1

Fiber 2.3

Carbs 3.5

Protein 2

94. Almonds and Oats Pudding

Preparation Time: 10 minutes

Cooking Time: 15 minutes

Servings: 4

Ingredients:

- 1 tablespoon lemon juice
- Zest of 1 lime
- 1 and ½ cups almond milk
- 1 teaspoon almond extract
- ½ cup oats
- 2 tablespoons stevia
- ½ cup silver almonds, chopped

Directions:

1. In a pan, combine the almond milk with the lime zest and the other ingredients, whisk, bring to a simmer and cook over medium heat for 15 minutes.
2. Divide the mix into bowls and serve cold.

Nutrition:

Calories 174 Fat 12.1

Fiber 3.2

Carbs 3.9

Protein 4.8

95. Strawberry Sorbet

Preparation Time: 15 minutes

Cooking Time: 10 minutes

Servings: 6

Ingredients:

- 1 cup strawberries, chopped
- 1 tablespoon of liquid honey
- 2 tablespoons water
- 1 tablespoon lemon juice

Directions:

1. Preheat the water and liquid honey until you get homogenous liquid.
2. Blend the strawberries until smooth and combine them with honey liquid and lemon juice.
3. Transfer the strawberry mixture in the ice cream maker and churn it for 20 minutes or until the sorbet is thick.
4. Scoop the cooked sorbet in the ice cream cups.

Nutrition:

Calories 30, Fat 0.4 g,

Fiber 1.4 g,

Carbs 14.9 g, Protein 0.9 g

96. Vanilla Apple Pie

Preparation Time: 15 minutes

Cooking Time: 50 minutes

Servings: 8

Ingredients:

- 3 apples, sliced
- ½ teaspoon ground cinnamon
- 1 teaspoon vanilla extract
- 1 tablespoon Erythritol
- 7 oz. yeast roll dough
- 1 egg, beaten

Directions:

1. Roll up the dough and cut it on 2 parts.
2. Line the springform pan with baking paper.
3. Place the first dough part in the springform pan.
4. Then arrange the apples over the dough and sprinkle it with Erythritol, vanilla extract, and ground cinnamon.
5. Then cover the apples with remaining dough and secure the edges of the pie with the help of the fork. Make the small cuts in the surface of the pie.
6. Brush the pie with beaten egg and bake it for 50 minutes at 375F.
7. Cool the cooked pie well and then remove from the springform pan. Cut it on the servings.

Nutrition:

Calories 140, Fat 3.4 g, Fiber 3.4 g, Carbs 23.9 g, Protein 2.9 g

97. Cinnamon Pears

Preparation Time: 2 hours

Cooking Time: 0 minutes

Servings: 6

Ingredients:

- 2 pears
- 1 teaspoon ground cinnamon
- 1 tablespoon Erythritol
- 1 teaspoon liquid stevia
- 4 teaspoons butter

Directions:

1. Cut the pears on the halves.
2. Then scoop the seeds from the pears with the help of the scooper.
3. In the shallow bowl mix up together Erythritol and ground cinnamon.
4. Sprinkle every pear half with cinnamon mixture and drizzle with liquid stevia.
5. Then add butter and wrap in the foil. Bake the pears for 25 minutes at 365F.
6. Then remove the pears from the foil and transfer in the serving plates.

Nutrition:

Calories 96, Fat 4.4 g, Fiber 1.4 g, Carbs 3.9 g, Protein 0.9 g

98. Ginger Ice Cream

Preparation Time: 15 minutes
Cooking Time: 10 minutes
Servings: 6
Ingredients:

- 1 mango, peeled
- 1 cup Greek yogurt
- 1 tablespoon Erythritol
- ¼ cup milk
- 1 teaspoon vanilla extract
- ¼ teaspoon ground ginger

Directions:

1. Blend the mango until you get puree and combine it with Erythritol, milk, vanilla extract, and ground ginger.
2. Then mix up together Greek yogurt and mango puree mixture. Transfer it in the plastic vessel.
3. Freeze the ice cream for 35 minutes.

Nutrition:

Calories 90, Fat 1.4 g, Fiber 1.4 g, Carbs 21.9 g, Protein 4.9 g

99. Cherry Compote

Preparation Time: 2 hours
Cooking Time: 0 minutes
Servings: 6
Ingredients:

- 2 peaches, pitted, halved
- 1 cup cherries, pitted
- ½ cup grape juice
- ½ cup strawberries
- 1 tablespoon liquid honey
- 1 teaspoon vanilla extract
- 1 teaspoon ground cinnamon

Directions:

1. Pour grape juice in the saucepan.
2. Add vanilla extract and ground cinnamon. Bring the liquid to boil.
3. After this, put peaches, cherries, and strawberries in the hot grape juice and bring to boil.
4. Remove the mixture from heat, add liquid honey, and close the lid.
5. Let the compote rest for 20 minutes.
6. Carefully mix up the compote and transfer in the serving plate.

Nutrition:

Calories 80, Fat 0.4 g, Fiber 2.4 g, Carbs 19.9 g, Protein 0.9 g

100.   Creamy Strawberries

Preparation Time: 15 minutes

Cooking Time: 10 minutes

Servings: 6

Ingredients:

- 6 tablespoons almond butter
- 1 tablespoon Erythritol
- 1 cup milk
- 1 teaspoon vanilla extract
- 1 cup strawberries, sliced

Directions:

1. Pour milk in the saucepan.
2. Add Erythritol, vanilla extract, and almond butter.
3. With the help of the hand mixer mix up the liquid until smooth and bring it to boil.
4. Then remove the mixture from the heat and let it cool.
5. The cooled mixture will be thick.
6. Put the strawberries in the serving glasses and top with the thick almond butter dip.

Nutrition:

Calories 192,

Fat 14.4 g,

Fiber 3.4 g,

Carbs 10.9 g,

Protein 1.9 g

CHAPTER 14:

Vegetables

101.   Buttered Carrot-Zucchini with Mayo

Preparation Time: 15 minutes

Cooking Time: 25 minutes

Servings: 4

Ingredients:

- 1 tablespoon grated onion
- 2 tablespoons butter, melted
- 1/2-pound carrots, sliced
- 1-1/2 zucchinis, sliced
- 1/4 cup water
- 1/4 cup mayonnaise
- 1/4 teaspoon prepared horseradish
- 1/4 teaspoon salt
- 1/4 teaspoon ground black pepper
- 1/4 cup Italian bread crumbs

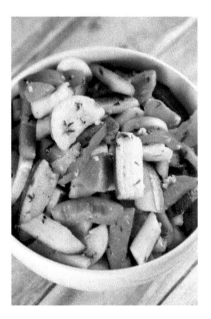

Directions:

1. Lighten skillet with cooking spray. Add the carrots. Cook for 360 minutes at 360oF. Add the zucchini and continue cooking for another 5 minutes.
2. Meanwhile, in a bowl, whisk together the pepper, salt, horseradish, onion, mayonnaise, and water. Pour into a vegetable skillet. Pull well over the coat.
3. In a small bowl, combine the melted butter and breadcrumbs. Sprinkle over the vegetables.
4. Cook for 10 minutes at 390oF until tops are lightly browned.
5. Serve and enjoy.

Nutrition:

Calories: 223

Carbs: 13.8g

Protein: 2.7g

Fat: 17.4g

102.   Tomato Bites with Creamy Parmesan Sauce

Preparation Time: 7 minutes

Cooking Time: 13 minutes

Servings: 4

Ingredients:

For the Sauce:

- 1/2 cup Parmigiano-Reggiano cheese, grated
- 4 tablespoons pecans, chopped
- 1 teaspoon garlic puree
- 1/2 teaspoon fine sea salt
- 1/3 cup extra-virgin olive oil

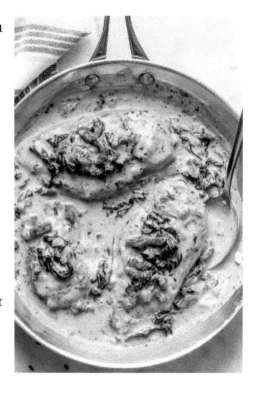

For the Tomato Bites:

- 2 large-sized Roma tomatoes, cut into thin slices and pat them dry
- 8 ounces Halloumi cheese, cut into thin slices
- 1/3 cup onions, sliced
- 1 teaspoon dried basil
- 1/4 teaspoon red pepper flakes, crushed
- 1/8 teaspoon sea salt

Directions:

1. Start by preheating your Air Fryer to 385 degrees F.
2. Make the sauce by mixing all ingredients, except the extra-virgin olive oil, in your food processor.
3. While the machine is running, slowly and gradually pour in the olive oil; puree until everything is well - blended.
4. Now, spread 1 teaspoon of the sauce over the top of each tomato slice. Place a slice of Halloumi cheese on each tomato slice. Top with onion slices. Sprinkle with basil, red pepper, and sea salt.
5. Transfer the assembled bites to the Air Fryer. Spray with non-stick cooking spray and cook for about 13 minutes.
6. Arrange these bites on a nice serving platter, garnish with the remaining sauce and serve at room temperature. Bon appétit!

Nutrition:

Calories: 428

Fat: 38.4g

Carbs: 4.5g

Protein: 18.8g

Sugars: 2.3g

Fiber: 1.3g

103.   Creamy Cauliflower and Broccoli

Preparation Time: 4 minutes

Cooking Time: 16 minutes

Servings: 6

Ingredients:

- 1-pound cauliflower florets
- 1-pound broccoli florets
- 2 ½ tablespoons sesame oil
- 1/2 teaspoon smoked cayenne pepper
- 3/4 teaspoon sea salt flakes
- 1 tablespoon lemon zest, grated
- 1/2 cup Colby cheese, shredded

Directions:

1. Prepare the cauliflower and broccoli using your favorite steaming method. Then, drain them well; add the sesame oil, cayenne pepper, and salt flakes.
2. Air-fry at 390 degrees F for approximately 16 minutes; make sure to check the vegetables halfway through the cooking time.
3. Afterwards, stir in the lemon zest and Colby cheese; toss to coat well and serve immediately!

Nutrition:

Calories: 133

Fat: 9.0g

Carbs: 9.5g

Protein: 5.9g

Sugars: 3.2g

Fiber: 3.6g

104. Mediterranean-Style Eggs with Spinach

Preparation Time: 3 minutes

Cooking Time: 12 minutes

Servings: 2

Ingredients:

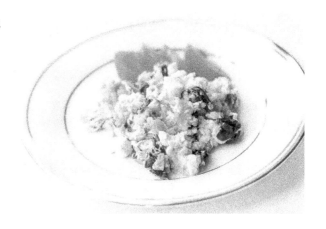

- 2 tablespoons olive oil, melted
- 4 eggs, whisked
- 5 ounces' fresh spinach, chopped
- 1 medium-sized tomato, chopped
- 1 teaspoon fresh lemon juice
- 1/2 teaspoon coarse salt
- 1/2 teaspoon ground black pepper
- 1/2 cup of fresh basil, roughly chopped

Directions:

1. Add the olive oil to an Air Fryer baking pan. Make sure to tilt the pan to spread the oil evenly.
2. Simply combine the remaining ingredients, except for the basil leaves; whisk well until everything is well incorporated.
3. Cook in the preheated oven for 8 to 12 minutes at 280 degrees F. Garnish with fresh basil leaves. Serve.

Nutrition:

Calories: 274

Fat: 23.2g

Carbs: 5.7g

Protein: 13.7g

Sugars: 2.6g

Fiber: 2.6g

105.   Spicy Zesty Broccoli with Tomato Sauce

Preparation Time: 5 minutes

Cooking Time: 15 minutes

Servings: 6

Ingredients:

For the Broccoli Bites:

- 1 medium-sized head broccoli, broken into florets
- 1/2 teaspoon lemon zest, freshly grated
- 1/3 teaspoon fine sea salt
- 1/2 teaspoon hot paprika
- 1 teaspoon shallot powder
- 1 teaspoon porcini powder
- 1/2 teaspoon granulated garlic
- 1/3 teaspoon celery seeds
- 1 ½ tablespoons olive oil

For the Hot Sauce:

- 1/2 cup tomato sauce
- 1 tablespoon balsamic vinegar
- ½ teaspoon ground allspice

Directions:

1. Toss all the ingredients for the broccoli bites in a mixing bowl, covering the broccoli florets on all sides.
2. Cook them in the preheated Air Fryer at 360 degrees for 13 to 15 minutes. In the meantime, mix all ingredients for the hot sauce.
3. Pause your Air Fryer, mix the broccoli with the prepared sauce and cook for a further 3 minutes. Bon appétit!

Nutrition:

Calories: 70

Fat: 3.8g

Carbs: 5.8g

Protein: 2g

Sugars: 6.6g

Fiber: 1.5g

106. Cheese Stuffed Mushrooms with Horseradish Sauce

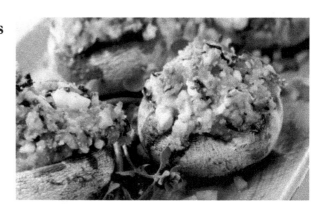

Preparation Time: 3 minutes

Cooking Time: 12 minutes

Servings: 5

Ingredients:

- 1/2 cup parmesan cheese, grated
- 2 cloves garlic, pressed
- 2 tablespoons fresh coriander, chopped
- 1/3 teaspoon kosher salt
- 1/2 teaspoon crushed red pepper flakes
- 1 ½ tablespoons olive oil
- 20 medium-sized mushrooms, cut off the stems
- 1/2 cup Gorgonzola cheese, grated
- 1/4 cup low-fat mayonnaise
- 1 teaspoon prepared horseradish, well-drained
- 1 tablespoon fresh parsley, finely chopped

Directions:

1. Mix the parmesan cheese together with the garlic, coriander, salt, red pepper, and the olive oil; mix to combine well.
2. Stuff the mushroom caps with the cheese filling. Top with grated Gorgonzola.
3. Place the mushrooms in the Air Fryer grill pan and slide them into the machine. Grill them at 380 degrees F for 8 to 12 minutes or until the stuffing is warmed through.
4. Meanwhile, prepare the horseradish sauce by mixing the mayonnaise, horseradish and parsley. Serve the horseradish sauce with the warm fried mushrooms. Enjoy!

Nutrition:

Calories: 180

Fat: 13.2g

Carbs: 6.2g

Protein: 8.6g

Sugars: 2.1g

Fiber: 1g

107.　　Tamarind Glazed Sweet Potatoes

Preparation Time: 2 minutes

Cooking Time: 22 minutes

Servings: 4

Ingredients:

- 1/3 teaspoon white pepper
- 1 tablespoon butter, melted
- 1/2 teaspoon turmeric powder
- 5 garnet sweet potatoes, peeled and diced
- A few drops liquid Stevia
- 2 teaspoons tamarind paste
- 1 1/2 tablespoons fresh lime juice
- 1 1/2 teaspoon ground allspice

Directions:

1. In a mixing bowl, toss all ingredients until sweet potatoes are well coated.
2. Air-fry them at 335 degrees F for 12 minutes.
3. Pause the Air Fryer and toss again. Increase the temperature to 390 degrees F and cook for an additional 10 minutes. Eat warm.

Nutrition:

Calories: 103

Fat: 9.1g

Carbs: 4.9g

Protein: 1.9g

Sugars: 1.2g

Fiber: 0.3g

108. Cauliflower Crust Pizza

Preparation Time: 20 minutes
Cooking Time: 45 minutes
Servings: 4

- **Ingredients:**
- I cauliflower (it should be cut into smaller portions)
- 1/4 grated parmesan cheese
- 1 egg
- 1 tsp. Italian seasoning
- 1/4 tsp. kosher salt
- 2 cups of freshly grated mozzarella
- 1/4 cup of spicy pizza sauce
- Basil leaves, for garnishing

Directions:

1. Begin by preheating your oven while using the parchment paper to rim the baking sheet.
2. Process the cauliflower into a fine powder, and then transfer to a bowl before putting it into the microwave.
3. Leave for about 5-6 minutes to get it soft.
4. Transfer the microwaved cauliflower to a clean and dry kitchen towel.
5. Leave it to cool off.
6. When cold, use the kitchen towel to wrap the cauliflower and then get rid of all the moisture by wringing the towel.
7. Continue squeezing until water is gone completely.
8. Put the cauliflower, Italian seasoning, Parmesan, egg, salt, and mozzarella (1 cup).
9. Stir very well until well combined.
10. Transfer the combined mixture to the baking sheet previously prepared, pressing it into a 10-inch round shape.
11. Bake for 10-15 minutes until it becomes golden in color.
12. Take the baked crust out of the oven and use the spicy pizza sauce and mozzarella (the leftover 1 cup) to top it.
13. Bake again for 10 more minutes until the cheese melts and looks bubbly.
14. Garnish using fresh basil leaves.
15. You can also enjoy this with salad.

Nutrition:

Calories: 74 Cal
Carbohydrates: 4 g
Protein: 6 g
Fat: 4 g
Fiber: 2 g

109.　　Thai Roasted Veggies

Preparation Time: 20 minutes
Cooking Time: 6 to 8 hours
Servings: 8
Ingredients:

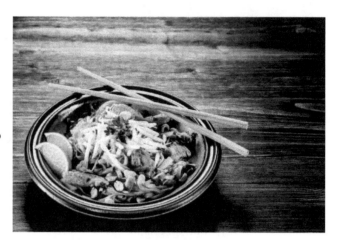

- 4 large carrots, peeled and cut into chunks
- 2 onions, peeled and sliced
- 6 garlic cloves, peeled and sliced
- 2 parsnips, peeled and sliced
- 2 jalapeño peppers, minced
- 1/2 cup Roasted Vegetable Broth
- 1/3 cup canned coconut milk
- 3 tablespoons lime juice
- 2 tablespoons grated fresh ginger root
- 2 teaspoons curry powder

Directions:

1. In a 6-quart slow cooker, mix the carrots, onions, garlic, parsnips, and jalapeño peppers.
2. In a small bowl, mix the vegetable broth, coconut milk, lime juice, ginger root, and curry powder until well blended. Pour this mixture into the slow cooker.
3. Cover and cook on low for 6 to 8 hours, do it until the vegetables are tender when pierced with a fork.

Nutrition:

Calories: 69 Cal

Carbohydrates: 13 g

Sugar: 6 g

Fiber: 3 g

Fat: 3g

Saturated Fat: 3g

Protein: 1g

Sodium: 95mg

110. Crispy-Topped Baked Vegetables

Preparation Time: 10 minutes
Cooking Time: 40 minutes
Servings: 4
Ingredients:

- 2 tbsp. olive oil
- 1 onion, chopped
- 1 celery stalk, chopped
- 2 carrots, grated
- 1/2-pound turnips, sliced
- 1 cup vegetable broth
- 1 tsp. turmeric
- Sea salt and black pepper, to taste
- 1/2 tsp. liquid smoke
- 1 cup Parmesan cheese, shredded
- 2 tbsp. fresh chives, chopped

Directions:

1. Set oven to 360°F and grease a baking dish with olive oil.
2. Set a skillet over medium heat and warm olive oil.
3. Sweat the onion until soft, and place in the turnips, carrots, and celery; and cook for 4 minutes.
4. Remove the vegetable mixture to the baking dish.
5. Combine vegetable broth with turmeric, pepper, liquid smoke, and salt.
6. Spread this mixture over the vegetables.
7. Sprinkle with Parmesan cheese and bake for about 30 minutes.
8. Garnish with chives to serve.

Nutrition:
Calories: 242 Cal
Fats: 16.3 g
Carbohydrates: 8.6 g
Protein: 16.3 g

111. Roasted Root Vegetables

Preparation Time: 20 minutes
Cooking Time: 6 to 8 hours
Servings: 8
Ingredients:

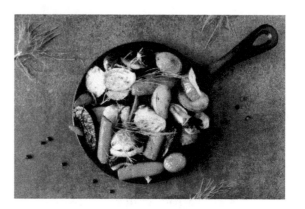

- 6 carrots, cut into 1-inch chunks
- 2 yellow onions, each cut into 8 wedges
- 2 sweet potatoes, peeled and cut into chunks
- 6 Yukon Gold potatoes, cut into chunks
- 8 whole garlic cloves, peeled
- 4 parsnips, peeled and cut into chunks
- 3 tablespoons olive oil
- 1 teaspoon dried thyme leaves
- 1/2 teaspoon salt
- 1/8 teaspoon freshly ground black pepper

Directions:

1. In a 6-quart slow cooker, mix all of the ingredients.
2. Cover and cook on low for 6 to 8 hours, or until the vegetables are tender.
3. Serve and enjoy!

Nutrition:

Calories: 214 Cal
Carbohydrates: 40 g
Sugar: 7 g
Fiber: 6 g
Fat: 5 g
Saturated Fat: 1 g
Protein: 4 g
Sodium: 201 mg

112.   HUMMUS

Preparation Time: 10 minutes

Cooking Time: 10 minutes

Servings: 32

Ingredients:

- 4 cups of cooked garbanzo beans
- 1 cup of water
- 11/2 tablespoons of lemon juice
- 2 teaspoons of ground cumin
- 11/2 teaspoon of ground coriander.
- 1 teaspoon of finely chopped garlic
- 1/2 teaspoon of salt
- 1/4 teaspoon of fresh ground pepper
- Paprika for garnish

Directions:

1. On a food processor, place together the garbanzo beans, lemon juice, water, garlic, salt, and pepper and process it until it becomes smooth and creamy.
2. To achieve your desired consistency, add more water.
3. Then spoon out the hummus in a serving bowl
4. Sprinkle your paprika and serve.

Nutrition:

Protein: 0.7 g

Carbohydrates: 2.5 g

Dietary Fiber: 0.6 g

Sugars: 0 g

Fat: 1.7 g

113.   Vegan Edamame Quinoa Collard Wraps

Preparation Time: 5 minutes
Cooking Time: 15 minutes
Servings: 4
Ingredients:
For the wrap:

- Collard leaves; 2 to 3
- Grated carrot; 1/4 cup
- Sliced cucumber; 1/4 cup
- Red bell pepper; 1/4; thin strips
- Orange bell pepper; 1/4; thin strips
- Cooked quinoa; 1/3 cup
- Shelled defrosted edamame; 1/3 cup

For the dressing:

- Fresh ginger root; 3 tablespoons; peeled and chopped
- Cooked chickpeas; 1 cup
- Clove of garlic; 1
- Rice vinegar; 4 tablespoons
- Low sodium tamari/coconut aminos; 2 tablespoons
- Lime juice; 2 tablespoons
- Water; 1/4 cup
- Few pinches of chili flakes
- Stevia; 1 pack

Directions:

1. For the dressing, combine all the ingredients and purée in a food processor until smooth.
2. Load into a little jar or tub, and set aside.
3. Place the collar leaves on a flat surface, covering one another to create a tighter tie.
4. Take one tablespoon of ginger dressing and blend it up with the prepared quinoa.
5. Spoon the prepared quinoa onto the leaves and shape a simple horizontal line at the closest end.
6. Supplement the edamame with all the veggie fillings left over.
7. Drizzle around one tablespoon of the ginger dressing on top, then fold the cover's sides inwards.
8. Pullover the fillings, the side of the cover closest to you, then turn the whole body away to seal it up.

Nutrition:
Calories: 295 Cal
Sugar: 3 g
Sodium: 200 mg
Fat: 13 g

CHAPTER 15:

Vegetables

114.   Cheesy Cauliflower Fritters

Difficulty: Medium
Preparation Time: 5 minutes
Cooking Time: 14 minutes
Servings: 8
Ingredients:

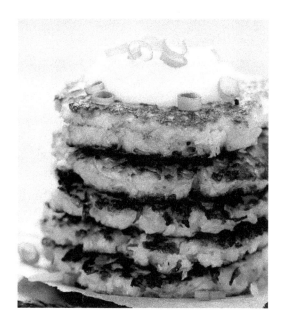

- ½ C. chopped parsley
- 1 C. Italian breadcrumbs
- 1/3 C. shredded mozzarella cheese
- 1/3 C. shredded sharp cheddar cheese
- 1 egg
- minced garlic cloves
- chopped scallions
- 1 head of cauliflower

Directions:

1   Cut cauliflower up into florets. Wash well and pat dry. Place into a food processor and pulse 20-30 seconds till it looks like rice.
2   Place cauliflower rice in a bowl and mix with pepper, salt, egg, cheeses, breadcrumbs, garlic, and scallions.
3   With hands, form 15 patties of the mixture. Add more breadcrumbs if needed.
4   With olive oil, spritz patties, and place into your air fryer in a single layer.
5   Cook 14 minutes at 390 degrees, flipping after 7 minutes.

Nutrition:

Calories: 209

Fat: 17g

Protein: 6g

Sugar: 0.5g

115.　　Avocado Fries

Difficulty: Medium
Preparation Time: 5 minutes
Cooking Time: 5 minutes
Servings: 6
Ingredients:

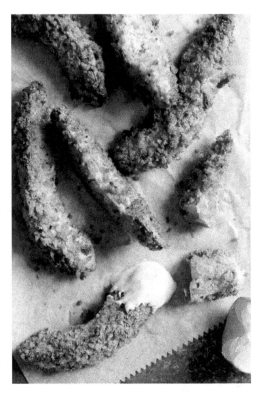

- 1 avocado
- ½ tsp. salt
- ½ C. panko breadcrumbs
- Bean liquid (aquafaba) from a 15-ounce can of white or garbanzo beans

Directions:

1　Peel, pit, and slice up avocado.
2　Toss salt and breadcrumbs together in a bowl. Place aquafaba into another bowl.
3　Dredge slices of avocado first in aquafaba and then in panko, making sure you get an even coating.
4　Place coated avocado slices into a single layer in the air fryer.
5　Cook 5 minutes at 390 degrees, shaking at 5 minutes.
6　Serve with your favorite dipping sauce!

Nutrition:

Calories: 102

Fat: 22g

Protein: 9g

Sugar: 1g

116.   Zucchini Parmesan Chips

Difficulty: Hard

Preparation Time: 5 minutes

Cooking Time: 8 minutes

Servings: 10

Ingredients:

- ½ tsp. paprika
- ½ C. grated parmesan cheese
- ½ C. Italian breadcrumbs
- 1 lightly beaten egg
- thinly sliced zucchinis

Directions:

1. Use a very sharp knife or mandolin slicer to slice zucchini as thinly as you can. Pat off extra moisture.
2. Beat egg with a pinch of pepper and salt and a bit of water.
3. Combine paprika, cheese, and breadcrumbs in a bowl.
4. Dip slices of zucchini into the egg mixture and then into breadcrumb mixture. Press gently to coat.
5. With olive oil cooking spray, mist coated zucchini slices. Place into your air fryer in a single layer.
6. Cook 8 minutes at 350 degrees.
7. Sprinkle with salt and serve with salsa.

Nutrition:

Calories: 211

Fat: 16g

Protein: 8g

Sugar: 0g

117.   Buffalo Cauliflower

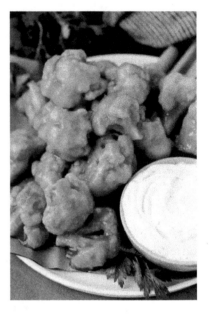

Difficulty: Hard

Preparation Time: 15 minutes

Cooking Time: 14 to 17 minutes

Servings: 6 to 8

Ingredients:

- Cauliflower:
- 1 C. panko breadcrumbs
- 1 tsp. salt
- C. cauliflower florets
- Buffalo Coating:
- ¼ C. Vegan Buffalo sauce
- ¼ C. melted vegan butter

Directions:

1   Melt butter in microwave and whisk in buffalo sauce.
2   Dip each cauliflower floret into buffalo mixture, ensuring it gets coated well. Hold over a bowl till floret is done dripping.
3   Mix breadcrumbs with salt.
4   Dredge dipped florets into breadcrumbs and place into air fryer.
5   Cook 14-17 minutes at 350 degrees. When slightly browned, they are ready to eat!
6   Serve with your favorite keto dipping sauce!

Nutrition:

Calories: 194

Fat: 17g

Protein: 10g

Sugar: 3g

118.   Air Fryer Brussels Sprouts

Difficulty: Hard

Preparation Time: 5 minutes

Cooking Time: 10 minutes

Servings: 5

Ingredients:

- ¼ tsp. salt
- 1 tbsp. balsamic vinegar
- 1 tbsp. olive oil
- C. Brussels sprouts

Directions:

1. Cut Brussels sprouts in half lengthwise. Toss with salt, vinegar, and olive oil till coated thoroughly.
2. Add coated sprouts to air fryer, cooking 8-10 minutes at 400 degrees. Shake after 5 minutes of cooking.
3. Brussels sprouts are ready to devour when brown and crisp!

Nutrition:

Calories: 118

Fat: 9g

Protein: 11g

Sugar: 1g

119.   Spaghetti Squash Tots

Difficulty: Hard

Preparation Time: 5 minutes

Cooking Time: 15 minutes

Servings: 8 to 10

Ingredients:

- ¼ tsp. pepper
- ½ tsp. salt
- 1 thinly sliced scallion
- 1 spaghetti squash

Directions:

1. Wash and cut the squash in half lengthwise. Scrape out the seeds.
2. With a fork, remove spaghetti meat by strands and throw out skins.
3. In a clean towel, toss in squash and wring out as much moisture as possible. Place in a bowl and with a knife slice through meat a few times to cut up smaller.
4. Add pepper, salt, and scallions to squash and mix well.
5. Create "tot" shapes with your hands and place in air fryer. Spray with olive oil.
6. Cook 15 minutes at 350 degrees until golden and crispy!

Nutrition:

Calories: 231 Fat: 18g Protein: 5g Sugar: 0g

120.   Cinnamon Butternut Squash Fries

Difficulty: Very Hard

Preparation Time: 10 minutes

Cooking Time: 10 minutes

Servings: 2

Ingredients:

- 1 pinch of salt
- 1 tbsp. powdered unprocessed sugar
- ½ tsp. nutmeg
- tsp. cinnamon
- 1 tbsp. coconut oil
- ounces pre-cut butternut squash fries

Directions:

1 In a plastic bag, pour in all ingredients. Coat fries with other components till coated and sugar is dissolved.
2 Spread coated fries into a single layer in the air fryer. Cook 10 minutes at 390 degrees until crispy.

Nutrition:

Calories: 175 Fat: 8g Protein: 1g Sugar: 5g

121.   Curried Cauliflower Florets

Difficulty: Very Hard

Preparation Time: 5 minutes

Cooking Time: 10 minutes

Servings: 4

Ingredients:

- 1/4 cup sultanas or golden raisins
- ¼ teaspoon salt
- 1 tablespoon curry powder
- 1 head cauliflower, broken into small florets
- ¼ cup pine nuts
- ½ cup olive oil

Directions:

1. In a cup of boiling water, soak your sultanas to plump. Preheat your air fryer to 350 degree Fahrenheit.
2. Add oil and pine nuts to air fryer and toast for a minute or so.
3. In a bowl toss the cauliflower and curry powder as well as salt, then add the mix to air fryer mixing well.
4. Cook for 10-minutes. Drain the sultanas, toss with cauliflower, and serve.

Nutrition:

Calories: 275, Total Fat: 11.3g, Carbs: 8.6g, Protein: 9.5g

122.   Oat and Chia Porridge

Difficulty: Very Hard

Preparation Time: 5 minutes

Cooking Time: 5 minutes

Servings: 4

Ingredients:

- tablespoons peanut butter
- teaspoons liquid Stevia
- 1 tablespoon butter, melted
- cups milk
- cups oats
- 1 cup chia seeds

Directions:

1 Preheat your air fryer to 390 degree Fahrenheit.
2 Whisk the peanut butter, butter, milk and Stevia in a bowl.
3 Stir in the oats and chia seeds.
4 Pour the mixture into an oven-proof bowl and place in the air fryer and cook for 5-minutes.

Nutrition:

Calories: 228, Total Fats: 11.4g,

Carbs: 10.2g, Protein: 14.5g

123.   Feta & Mushroom Frittata

Difficulty: Very Hard

Preparation Time: 15 minutes

Cooking Time: 30 minutes

Servings: 4

Ingredients:

- 1 red onion, thinly sliced
- cups button mushrooms, thinly sliced
- Salt to taste
- tablespoons feta cheese, crumbled
- medium eggs
- Non-stick cooking spray
- tablespoons olive oil

Directions:

1 Saute the onion and mushrooms in olive oil over medium heat until the vegetables are tender.
2   Remove the vegetables from pan and drain on a paper towel-lined plate.
3   In a mixing bowl, whisk eggs and salt. Coat all sides of baking dish with cooking spray.
4   Preheat your air fryer to 325 degree Fahrenheit. Pour the beaten eggs into prepared baking dish and scatter the sautéed vegetables and crumble feta on top. Bake in the air fryer for 30-minutes. Allow to cool slightly and serve!

Nutrition:

Calories: 226, Total Fat: 9.3g, Carbs: 8.7g, Protein: 12.6g

124.   Butter Glazed Carrots

Difficulty: Very Hard

Preparation Time: 20 Minutes

Cooking Time: 15 minutes

Servings: 4

Ingredients:

- Baby carrots-2 cups
- Brown sugar-1 tbsps.
- Butter; melted-1/2 tbsps.
- Salt and black pepper- a pinch

Directions:

1 Take a baking dish suitable to fit in your air fryer.
2 Toss carrots with sugar, butter, salt and black peppers in that baking dish.
3 Place this dish in the air fryer basket and seal the fryer.
4 Cook the carrots for 10 minutes at 3500 F on Air fryer mode.
5 Enjoy.

Nutrition:

Calories 151,

Fat 2,

Fiber 4,

Carbs 14,

Protein 4

CHAPTER 16:

Sauces, Soup and Stew Recipes

125.   Cranberry Sauce

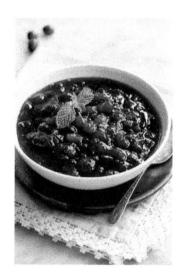

Preparation Time: 5 minutes
Cooking Time: 8 minutes
Servings: 2
Ingredients:

- ¾ cup fresh cranberries
- 2 tbsp. raw honey
- ½ cup pure squeezed orange juice
- ½ tsp. cinnamon
- 1 tbsp. stevia

Directions:

1. Put all the **Ingredients:** in the Instant Pot.
2. Secure the lid and turn the pressure release handle to the "sealed" position.
3. Select the MANUAL functions, set to HIGH PRESSURE, and adjust the timer to 8 minutes.
4. After the beep, "QUICK-RELEASE" the steam and remove the lid.
5. Serve when cool, or save in a bottle for later use.

Nutrition:

Calories: 62

Fat: 0 g

Carbohydrate: 17 g

Protein: 0.1 g

126.   Béarnaise Sauce

Preparation Time: 5 minutes
Cooking Time: 3 minutes
Servings: 2
Ingredients:

- ½ cup butter
- 2 egg yolks, beaten
- 2 tsp. lemon juice, freshly squeezed
- ¼ tsp. onion powder
- 2 tbsp. fresh tarragon

Directions:

1. Press the SAUTÉ button on the Instant Pot.
2. Melt the butter for 3 minutes and transfer it into a mixing bowl.
3. While whisking the melted butter, slowly add the egg yolks.
4. Continue stirring so that no lumps form.
5. Add the lemon juice, onion powder, and fresh tarragon.
6. Serve.

Nutrition:

Calories: 603
Fat: 62 g
Carbs: 4 g
Protein: 5 g

127.   Chili Sauce

Preparation Time: 8 minutes
Cooking Time: 15 minutes
Servings: 2
Ingredients:

- 2 oz. hot peppers
- 2 cups of apple cider vinegar
- 1 tsp. salt

Directions:

1. Trim away the stems from the peppers and chop.
2. Add all **Ingredients:** to the Instant Pot.
3. Secure the lid and MANUALLY set the timer to 15 minutes under HIGH pressure.
4. Quick-release the pressure and serve the sauce into bowls.

Nutrition:

Calories: 2
Fat: 0 g
Carbs: 0.7 g
Protein: 1 g

128. Vanilla Caramel Sauce

Preparation Time: 5 minutes

Cooking Time: 13 minutes

Servings: 2

Ingredients:

- 2 tbsp. coconut oil
- 1 cup sugar
- 1 tsp vanilla extract
- 1/3 cup condensed coconut milk
- 1/3 cup water

Directions:

1. Warm up the Instant Pot using the SAUTÉ function.
2. Add the water and sugar, then stir and sauté for 13 minutes.
3. Stir in the milk, coconut oil, and vanilla.
4. Whisk until creamy and add to a glass container. Cool completely and serve when ready.

Nutrition:

Calories: 80 Carbs: 14 g Fat: 5 g Protein: 0 g

129. Delicious Chicken Soup

Preparation Time: 10 minutes

Cooking Time: 4 hours 30 minutes

Servings: 4

Ingredients:

- 1 lb. chicken breasts, boneless and skinless
- 2 Tbsp. fresh basil, chopped
- 1 1/2 cups mozzarella cheese, shredded
- 2 garlic cloves, minced
- 1 Tbsp. Parmesan cheese, grated
- 2 Tbsp. dried basil
- 2 cups chicken stock
- 28 oz. tomatoes, diced
- 1/4 tsp pepper
- 1/2 tsp salt

Directions:

1. Add chicken, Parmesan cheese, dried basil, tomatoes, garlic, pepper, and salt to a crock pot and stir well to combine. Cover and cook on low for 4 hours.
2. Add fresh basil and mozzarella cheese and stir well.
3. Cover again and cook for 30 more minutes or until cheese is melted.
4. Remove chicken from the crock pot and shred using forks. Return shredded chicken to the crock pot and stir to mix. Serve and enjoy.

Nutrition:

Calories 299 Fat 16 g Carbohydrates 3 g Sugar 6 g Protein 38 g Cholesterol 108 mg

130.   Flavorful Broccoli Soup

Preparation Time: 10 minutes

Cooking Time: 4 hours 15 minutes

Servings: 6

Ingredients:

- 20 oz. broccoli florets
- 4 oz. cream cheese
- 8 oz. cheddar cheese, shredded
- 1/2 tsp paprika
- 1/2 tsp ground mustard
- 3 cups chicken stock
- 2 garlic cloves, chopped
- 1 onion, diced
- 1 cup carrots, shredded
- 1/4 tsp baking soda
- 1/4 tsp salt

Directions:

1. Add all ingredients except cream cheese and cheddar cheese to a crock pot and stir well.
2. Cover and cook on low for 4 hours.
3. Purée the soup using an immersion blender until smooth.
4. Stir in the cream cheese and cheddar cheese.
5. Cover and cook on low for 15 minutes longer.
6. Season with pepper and salt.
7. Serve and enjoy.

Nutrition:

Calories 275

Fat 19 g

Carbohydrates 19 g

Sugar 4 g

Protein 14 g

Cholesterol 60 mg

131. Healthy Spinach Soup

Preparation Time: 10 minutes

Cooking Time: 3 hours

Servings: 8

Ingredients:

- 3 cups frozen spinach, chopped, thawed and drained
- 8 oz. cheddar cheese, shredded
- 1 egg, lightly beaten
- 10 oz. can cream of chicken soup
- 8 oz. cream cheese, softened

Directions:

1. Add spinach to a large bowl. Purée the spinach.
2. Add egg, chicken soup, cream cheese, and pepper to the spinach purée and mix well.
3. Transfer spinach mixture to a crock pot.
4. Cover and cook on low for 3 hours.
5. Stir in cheddar cheese and serve.

Nutrition:

Calories 256

Fat 29 g

Carbohydrates 1 g

Sugar 0.5 g

Protein 11 g

Cholesterol 84 mg

132.   Healthy Chicken Kale Soup

Preparation Time: 10 minutes
Cooking Time: 6 hours 15 minutes
Servings: 6
Ingredients:

- 2 lb. chicken breasts, skinless and boneless
- 1/4 cup fresh lemon juice
- 5 oz. baby kale
- 32 oz. chicken stock
- 1/2 cup olive oil
- 1 large onion, sliced
- 14 oz. chicken broth
- 1 Tbsp. extra-virgin olive oil
- Salt

Directions:

1. Heat the extra-virgin olive oil in a pan over medium heat.
2. Season chicken with salt and place in the hot pan.
3. Cover pan and cook chicken for 15 minutes.
4. Remove chicken from the pan and shred it using forks.
5. Add shredded chicken to a crock pot.
6. Add sliced onion, olive oil, and broth to a blender and blend until combined.
7. Pour blended mixture into the crock pot.
8. Add remaining ingredients to the crock pot and stir well.
9. Cover and cook on low for 6 hours.
10. Stir well and serve.

Nutrition:
Calories 493
Fat 33 g
Carbohydrates 8 g
Sugar 9 g
Protein 47 g
Cholesterol 135 mg

133.   Spicy Chicken Pepper Stew

Preparation Time: 10 minutes

Cooking Time: 6 hours

Servings: 6

Ingredients:

- 3 chicken breasts, skinless and boneless, cut into small pieces
- 1 tsp garlic, minced
- 1 tsp ground ginger
- 2 tsp olive oil
- 2 tsp soy sauce
- 1 Tbsp. fresh lemon juice
- 1/2 cup green onions, sliced
- 1 Tbsp. crushed red pepper
- 8 oz. chicken stock
- 1 bell pepper, chopped
- 1 green chili pepper, sliced
- 2 jalapeño peppers, sliced
- 1/2 tsp black pepper
- 1/4 tsp sea salt

Directions:

1. Add all ingredients to a large mixing bowl and mix well. Place in the refrigerator overnight.
2. Pour marinated chicken mixture into a crock pot.
3. Cover and cook on low for 6 hours.
4. Stir well and serve.

Nutrition:

Calories 171

Fat 4 g

Carbohydrates 7 g

Sugar 7 g

Protein 22 g

Cholesterol 65 mg

134.   Creamy Broccoli Cauliflower Soup

Preparation Time: 10 minutes

Cooking Time: 6 hours

Servings: 6

Ingredients:

- 2 cups cauliflower florets, chopped
- 3 cups broccoli florets, chopped
- 3 1/2 cups chicken stock
- 1 large carrot, diced
- 1/2 cup shallots, diced
- 2 garlic cloves, minced
- 1 cup plain yogurt
- 6 oz. cheddar cheese, shredded
- 1 cup coconut milk
- Pepper
- Salt

Directions:

1. Add all ingredients except milk, cheese, and yogurt to a crock pot and stir well.
2. Cover and cook on low for 6 hours.
3. Purée the soup using an immersion blender until smooth.
4. Add cheese, milk, and yogurt and blend until smooth and creamy.
5. Season with pepper and salt.
6. Serve and enjoy.

Nutrition:

Calories 281

Fat 20 g

Carbohydrates 14 g

Sugar 9 g

Protein 11 g

Cholesterol 32 mg

135. Mexican Chicken Soup

Preparation Time: 10 minutes
Cooking Time: 4 hours
Servings: 6
Ingredients:

- 1 1/2 lb. chicken thighs, skinless and boneless
- 14 oz. chicken stock
- 14 oz. salsa
- 8 oz. Monterey Jack cheese, shredded

Directions:

1. Place chicken into a crock pot.
2. Pour remaining ingredients over the chicken.
3. Cover and cook on high for 4 hours.
4. Remove chicken from crock pot and shred using forks.
5. Return shredded chicken to the crock pot and stir well.
6. Serve and enjoy.

Nutrition:

Calories 371

Fat 15 g

Carbohydrates 7 g

Sugar 2 g

Protein 41 g

Cholesterol 135 mg

136.   Beef Stew

Preparation Time: 10 minutes
Cooking Time: 5 hours 5 minutes
Servings: 8
Ingredients:

- 3 lb. beef stew meat, trimmed
- 1/2 cup red curry paste
- 1/3 cup tomato paste
- 13 oz. can coconut milk
- 2 tsp ginger, minced
- 2 garlic cloves, minced
- 1 medium onion, sliced
- 2 Tbsp. olive oil
- 2 cups carrots, julienned
- 2 cups broccoli florets
- 2 tsp fresh lime juice
- 2 Tbsp. fish sauce
- 2 tsp sea salt

Directions:

1. Heat 1 tablespoon of oil in a pan over medium heat.
2. Brown the meat on all sides in the pan.
3. Add brown meat to a crock pot.
4. Add remaining oil to the same pan and sauté the ginger, garlic, and onion over medium-high heat for 5 minutes.
5. Add coconut milk and stir well.
6. Transfer pan mixture to the crock pot.
7. Add remaining ingredients except for carrots and broccoli.
8. Cover and cook on high for 5 hours.
9. Add carrots and broccoli during the last 30 minutes of cooking.
10. Serve and enjoy.

Nutrition:

Calories 537

Fat 26 g

Carbohydrates 13 g

Sugar 16 g

Protein 54 g

Cholesterol 152 mg

137.   Tasty Basil Tomato Soup

Preparation Time: 10 minutes
Cooking Time: 6 hours
Servings: 6
Ingredients:

- 28 oz. can whole peeled tomatoes
- 1/2 cup fresh basil leaves
- 4 cups chicken stock
- 1 tsp red pepper flakes
- 3 garlic cloves, peeled
- 2 onions, diced
- 3 carrots, peeled and diced
- 3 Tbsp. olive oil
- 1 tsp salt

Directions:

1. Add all ingredients to a crock pot and stir well.
2. Cover and cook on low for 6 hours.
3. Purée the soup until smooth using an immersion blender.
4. Season soup with pepper and salt.
5. Serve and enjoy.

Nutrition:

Calories 126

Fat 5 g

Carbohydrates 13 g

Sugar 7 g

Protein 5 g

Cholesterol 0 mg

138.   Beef Chili

Preparation Time: 10 minutes
Cooking Time: 8 hours
Servings: 6
Ingredients:

- 1 lb. ground beef
- 1 tsp garlic powder
- 1 tsp paprika
- 3 tsp chili powder
- 1 Tbsp. Worcestershire sauce
- 1 Tbsp. fresh parsley, chopped
- 1 tsp onion powder
- 25 oz. tomatoes, chopped
- 4 carrots, chopped
- 1 onion, diced
- 1 bell pepper, diced
- 1/2 tsp sea salt

Directions:

1. Brown the ground meat in a pan over high heat until meat is no longer pink.
2. Transfer meat to a crock pot.
3. Add bell pepper, tomatoes, carrots, and onion to the crock pot and stir well.
4. Add remaining ingredients and stir well.
5. Cover and cook on low for 8 hours.
6. Serve and enjoy.

Nutrition:

Calories 152
Fat 4 g
Carbohydrates 4 g
Sugar 8 g
Protein 18 g
Cholesterol 51 mg

CHAPTER 17:

Seafood

139.   Mozzarella Fish

Preparation Time: 5 minutes

Cooking Time: 10-15 minutes

Servings: 6-8

Ingredients:

- 2 lbs. of bone gold sole
- Salt and pepper to taste
- ½ teaspoon dried oregano
- 1 cup grated mozzarella cheese
- 1 large fresh tomato, sliced thinly

Directions:

1. Excellent source of cooking the butter. Organize a single layer of trout. Add salt, pepper, and oregano.
2. Top with sliced cheese slices and tomatoes.
3. Cook, covered, for 10 to 15 minutes at 425°F.

Nutrition:

Calories: 156 Fat: 6g Net Carbs: 5g Protein: 8g

140.   Cucumber Ginger Shrimp

Preparation Time: 5 minutes

Cooking Time: 10 minutes

Servings: 1

Ingredients:

- 1 large cucumber, sliced into 1/2-inch round
- 10-15 large shrimp/prawns
- 1 teaspoon (1 g) fresh ginger, grated
- Salt to taste
- Coconut oil to cook with

Directions:

1. Pour 1 Tablespoon (15 ml) of coconut oil into a frying pan on medium heat.
2. Put the ginger and the cucumber and sauté for 2-3 minutes.
3. Add in the shrimp then cook until they turn pink and are no longer translucent.
4. Add salt to taste and serve.

Nutrition:

Calories: 250 Fat: 16 g Net Carbohydrates: 4 g Protein: 20 g

141. Salmon with Pesto

Preparation Time: 10 minutes
Cooking Time: 15 minutes
Servings: 4
Ingredients:

- 4 salmon fillets
- 2 teaspoons olive oil
- Pinch of salt
- ½-cup pesto

Directions:

1. Arrange the greased Cook & Crisp Basket in the pot of Ninja Foodi.
2. Close the Ninja Foodi with crisping lid and select Air Crisp.
3. Set the temperature to 270 degrees F for 5 minutes.
4. Press Start/Stop to begin preheating.
5. Drizzle the salmon fillets with oil evenly and sprinkle with a pinch of salt.
6. After preheating, open the lid.
7. Place the salmon fillets into the Cook & Crisp Basket.
8. Close the Ninja Foodi with crisping lid and select Air Crisp.
9. Set the temperature to 270 degrees F for 20 minutes.
10. Press Start/Stop to begin cooking. Transfer the salmon fillets onto a platter and top with the pesto.
11. Serve immediately.

Nutrition:

Calories: 380 Fats: 25.8g Carbohydrates: 2g Proteins: 36g

142. Salmon in Dill Sauce

Preparation Time: 10 minutes
Cooking Time: 2 hours
Servings: 6
Ingredients:

- 2 cups water
- 1-cup homemade chicken broth
- 2 tablespoons fresh lemon juice
- ¼ cup fresh dill, chopped
- 6 salmon fillets
- 1 teaspoon cayenne pepper
- Salt and ground black pepper

Directions:

1. In the pot of Ninja Foodi, mix together the water, broth, lemon juice, lemon juice and dill.
2. Organize the salmon fillets on top, skin side down, and sprinkle with cayenne pepper, salt black pepper.
3. Close the Ninja Foodi with crisping lid and select Slow Cooker.
4. Set on Low for 1-2 hours. Press Start/Stop to begin cooking. Serve hot.

Nutrition:

Calories: 164 Fats: 7.4g Carbohydrates 1.6 g Proteins: 23.3g

143. Seasoned Catfish

Preparation Time: 15 minutes

Cooking Time: 23 minutes

Servings: 4

Ingredients:

- 4 catfish fillets
- 2 tablespoons Italian seasoning
- Salt and ground black pepper
- 1 tablespoon olive oil
- 1 tablespoon fresh parsley, chopped

Directions:

1. Arrange the greased Cook & Crisp Basket in the pot of Ninja Foodi.
2. Close the Ninja Foodi with crisping lid and select Air Crisp.
3. Set the temperature to 400 °F for 5 minutes.
4. Press Start/Stop to begin preheating.
5. Rub the fish fillets with seasoning, salt, and black pepper generously and then coat with oil.
6. After preheating, open the lid.
7. Place the catfish fillets into the Cook & Crisp Basket.
8. Close the Ninja Foodi with crisping lid and select Air Crisp.
9. Set the temperature to 400°F for 20 minutes. Press Start/Stop to begin cooking. Flip the fish fillets once halfway through. Serve hot with the garnishing of parsley.

Nutrition:

Calories: 205 Fats: 14.2g Carbohydrates 0.8 g Proteins: 17.7g

144. Parsley Tilapia

Preparation Time: 15 minutes

Cooking Time: 1 hour and 30 minutes

Servings: 6

Ingredients:

- 6 tilapia fillets
- Salt and ground black pepper
- ½ cup yellow onion, chopped
- 3 teaspoons fresh lemon rind, grated finely
- ¼ cup fresh parsley, chopped
- 2 tablespoon unsalted butter, melted

Directions:

1. Grease the pot of Ninja Foodi.
2. Spice the tilapia fillets with salt and black pepper generously.
3. In the prepared pot of Ninja Foodi, place the tilapia fillets.
4. Arrange the onion, lemon rind, and parsley over fillets evenly and drizzle with melted butter.
5. Close the Ninja Foodi with crisping lid and select Slow Cooker. Set on Low for 1½ hours.
6. Press Start/Stop to begin cooking. Serve hot.

Nutrition:

Calories: 133 Fats: 4.9g Carbohydrates: 1.3g Proteins: 21.3g

145.   Crispy Tilapia

Preparation Time: 15 minutes

Cooking Time: 14 minutes

Servings: 4

Ingredients:

- ¾ cup pork rinds, crushed
- 1 packet dry ranch-style dressing mix
- 2½ tablespoons olive oil
- 2 organic eggs
- 4 tilapia fillets

Directions:

1. Arrange the greased Cook & Crisp Basket in the pot of Ninja Foodi.
2. Close the Ninja Foodi with crisping lid and select Air Crisp.
3. Set the temperature to 355 degrees F for 5 minutes.
4. Press "Start/Stop" to begin preheating.
5. In a shallow bowl, beat the eggs.
6. In another bowl, add the pork rinds, ranch dressing, and oil and mix until a crumbly mixture form.
7. Put the fish fillets into the egg then coat with the pork rind mixture.
8. After preheating, open the lid.
9. Arrange the tilapia fillets in the prepared Cook & Crisp Basket in a single layer.
10. Close the Ninja Foodi with crisping lid and select Air Crisp.
11. Set the temperature to 350°F for 14 minutes.
12. Press Start/Stop to begin cooking.
13. Serve hot.

Nutrition:

Calories: 304

Fats: 16.8g

 Carbohydrates 0.4 g

 Proteins: 38g

146.   Cod with Tomatoes

Preparation Time: 15 minutes

Cooking Time: 16 minutes

Servings: 4

Ingredients:

- 1-pound cherry tomatoes halved
- 2 tablespoons fresh rosemary, chopped
- 4 cod fillets
- 2 garlic cloves, minced
- 1 tablespoon olive oil
- Salt and ground black pepper

Directions:

1. At the bottom of a greased a large heatproof bowl, place half of the cherry tomatoes followed by the rosemary.
2. Arrange cod fillets on top in a single layer, followed by the remaining tomatoes.
3. Sprinkle with garlic and drizzle with oil.
4. At the bottom of Ninja Foodie, arrange the bowl.
5. Close the Ninja Foodi with the pressure lid and place the pressure valve to Seal position.
6. Select Pressure and set to High for 6 minutes.
7. Press Start/Stop to begin cooking.
8. Switch the valve to Vent and do a quick release.
9. Transfer the fish fillets and tomatoes onto serving plates.
10. Sprinkle with salt and black pepper and serve.

Nutrition:

Calories: 149

Fats: 5g

Carbohydrates 6 g

Proteins: 21.4g

147.   Crab Casserole

Preparation Time: 10 minutes
Cooking Time: 30 minutes
Servings: 5
Ingredients:

- 2 tbsp. of oil, for frying
- 1 onion, finely chopped
- 150 g finely chopped celery stalks
- salt and pepper
- 300 ml homemade mayonnaise
- 4 eggs
- 450 g canned crab meat
- 325 g grated white cheddar cheese
- 2 tsp. paprika
- ¼ tsp. cayenne pepper
- For filing
- 75 g leafy greens
- 2 tbsp. of olive oil

Directions:

1. Set the oven to 350°F. Grease a 9x12 baking dish.
2. Fry onion and celery in oil until translucent.
3. In another bowl, add mayonnaise, eggs, crab meat, seasonings, and ⅔ chopped cheese. Add the fried onions and celery and stir.
4. Add the mass to the baking dish. Sprinkle the remaining cheese on top and bake for about 30 minutes or until golden brown.
5. Serve with salad and olive oil.

Nutrition:

Carbohydrates: 6 g

Fats: 95 g

Proteins: 47 g

Calories: 400

148.   Cod with Bell Pepper

Preparation Time: 15 minutes

Cooking Time: 1 hour and 30 minutes

Servings: 4

Ingredients:

- 1 bell pepper, seeded and sliced
- ½ small onion, sliced
- 3 garlic cloves, minced
- 1 can sugar-free diced tomatoes
- 1 tablespoon fresh rosemary, chopped
- ¼ cup homemade fish broth
- ¼ teaspoon red pepper flakes
- Salt and ground black pepper
- 1-pound cod fillets

Directions:

1. In the pot of Ninja Foodi, add all the ingredients except cod and stir to combine.
2. Season cod fillets with salt and black pepper evenly.
3. Arrange the cod fillets over broth mixture.
4. Close the Ninja Foodi with crisping lid and select Slow Cooker.
5. Set on High for 1½ hours.
6. Press Start/Stop to begin cooking.
7. Serve hot.

Nutrition:

Calories: 129

Fats: 1.6g

Carbohydrates 7.7 g

Proteins: 22.1g

149.   Shrimp with Garlic

Preparation Time: 10 minutes
Cooking Time: 25 minutes
Servings: 2
Ingredients:

- 1 lb. shrimp
- ¼ teaspoon baking soda
- 2 tablespoons oil
- 2 teaspoon minced garlic
- ¼ cup vermouth
- 2 tablespoons unsalted butter
- 1 teaspoon parsley

Directions:

1. In a bowl toss shrimp with baking soda and salt, let it stand for a couple of minutes
2. In a skillet heat olive oil and add shrimp
3. Add garlic, red pepper flakes and cook for 1-2 minutes
4. Add vermouth and cook for another 4-5 minutes
5. When ready remove from heat and serve

Nutrition:

Calories: 289
Total Carbohydrate: 2 g
Cholesterol: 3 mg
Total Fat: 17 g
Fiber: 2 g
Protein: 7 g
Sodium: 163 mg

150.   Sabich Sandwich

Preparation Time: 5 minutes
Cooking Time: 15 minutes
Servings: 2
Ingredients:

- 2 tomatoes
- Olive oil
- ½ lb. eggplant
- ¼ cucumber
- 1 tablespoon lemon
- 1 tablespoon parsley
- ¼ head cabbage
- 2 tablespoons wine vinegar
- 2 pita bread
- ½ cup hummus
- ¼ tahini sauce
- 2 hard-boiled eggs

Directions:

1. In a skillet fry eggplant slices until tender
2. In a bowl add tomatoes, cucumber, parsley, lemon juice and season salad
3. In another bowl toss cabbage with vinegar
4. In each pita pocket add hummus, eggplant and drizzle tahini sauce
5. Top with eggs, tahini sauce

Nutrition:

Calories: 269
Total Carbohydrate: 2 g
Cholesterol: 3 mg
Total Fat: 14 g
Fiber: 2 g
Protein: 7 g
Sodium: 183 mg

151.   Salmon with Vegetables

Preparation Time: 10 minutes

Cooking Time: 15 minutes

Servings: 4

Ingredients:

- 2 tablespoons olive oil
- 2 carrots
- 1 head fennel
- 2 squash
- ¼ onion
- 1-inch ginger
- 1 cup white wine
- 2 cups water
- 2 parsley sprigs
- 2 tarragon sprigs
- 6 oz. salmon fillets
- 1 cup cherry tomatoes
- 1 scallion

Directions:

1. In a skillet heat olive oil, add fennel, squash, onion, ginger, carrot and cook until vegetables are soft
2. Add wine, water, parsley and cook for another 4-5 minutes
3. Season salmon fillets and place in the pan
4. Cook for 5 minutes per side or until is ready
5. Transfer salmon to a bowl, spoon tomatoes and scallion around salmon and serve

Nutrition:

Calories: 301

Total Carbohydrate: 2 g

Cholesterol: 13 mg

Total Fat: 17 g

Fiber: 4 g

Protein: 8 g

Sodium: 201 mg

152. Moules Marinieres

Preparation Time: 10 minutes

Cooking Time: 30 minutes

Servings: 4

Ingredients:

- 2 tablespoons unsalted butter
- 1 leek
- 1 shallot
- 2 cloves garlic
- 2 bay leaves
- 1 cup white win
- 2 lb. mussels
- 2 tablespoons mayonnaise
- 1 tablespoon lemon zest
- 2 tablespoons parsley
- 1 sourdough bread

Directions:

1. In a saucepan melt butter, add leeks, garlic, bay leaves, shallot and cook until vegetables are soft
2. Bring to a boil, add mussels, and cook for 1-2 minutes
3. Transfer mussels to a bowl and cover
4. Whisk in remaining butter with mayonnaise and return mussels to pot
5. Add lemon juice, parsley lemon zest and stir to combine

Nutrition:

Calories: 321

Total Carbohydrate: 2 g

Cholesterol: 13 mg

Total Fat: 17 g

Fiber: 2 g

Protein: 9 g

Sodium: 312 mg

153.   Steamed Mussels with Coconut-Curry

Preparation Time: 15 minutes

Cooking Time: 20 minutes

Servings: 4

Ingredients:

- 6 sprigs cilantro
- 2 cloves garlic
- 2 shallots
- ¼ teaspoon coriander seeds
- ¼ teaspoon red chili flakes
- 1 teaspoon zest
- 1 can coconut milk
- 1 tablespoon vegetable oil
- 1 tablespoon curry paste
- 1 tablespoon brown sugar
- 1 tablespoon fish sauce
- 2 lb. mussels

Directions:

1. In a bowl combine lime zest, cilantro stems, shallot, garlic, coriander seed, chili and salt
2. In a saucepan heat oil add, garlic, shallots, pounded paste and curry paste
3. Cook for 3-4 minutes, add coconut milk, sugar and fish sauce
4. Bring to a simmer and add mussels
5. Stir in lime juice, cilantro leaves and cook for a couple of more minutes
6. When ready remove from heat and serve

Nutrition:

Calories: 209

Total Carbohydrate: 6 g

Cholesterol: 13 mg

Total Fat: 7 g

Fiber: 2 g

Protein: 17 g

Sodium: 193 mg

154. Salmon Burgers

Preparation Time: 10 minutes
Cooking Time: 15 minutes
Servings: 4
Ingredients:

- 1 lb. salmon fillets
- 1 onion
- ¼ dill fronds
- 1 tablespoon honey
- 1 tablespoon horseradish
- 1 tablespoon mustard
- 1 tablespoon olive oil
- 2 toasted split rolls
- 1 avocado

Directions:

1. Place salmon fillets in a blender and blend until smooth, transfer to a bowl, add onion, dill, honey, horseradish and mix well
2. Add salt and pepper and form 4 patties
3. In a bowl combine mustard, honey, mayonnaise and dill
4. In a skillet heat oil add salmon patties and cook for 2-3 minutes per side
5. When ready remove from heat
6. Divided lettuce and onion between the buns
7. Place salmon patty on top and spoon mustard mixture and avocado slices
8. Serve when ready

Nutrition:

Calories: 189

Total Carbohydrate: 6 g

Cholesterol: 3 mg

Total Fat: 7 g

Fiber: 4 g

Protein: 12 g

Sodium: 293 mg

CHAPTER 18:

Meat

155.   Beef with Carrot & Broccoli

Preparation Time: 15 minutes

Cooking Time: 14 minutes

Servings: 4

Ingredients:

- 2 tbsp. coconut oil, divided
- 2 medium garlic cloves, minced
- 1 lb. beef sirloin steak, sliced into thin strips
- Salt, to taste
- ¼ cup chicken broth
- 2 tsp. fresh ginger, grated
- 1 tbsp. Ground flax seeds
- ½ tsp. Red pepper flakes, crushed
- ¼ tsp. freshly ground black pepper
- 1 large carrot, peeled and sliced thinly
- 2 cups broccoli florets
- 1 medium scallion, sliced thinly

Directions:

1. In a skillet, warm 1 tbsp. of oil on medium-high heat.
2. Put garlic and sauté approximately 1 minute.
3. Add beef and salt and cook for at least 4-5 minutes or till browned.
4. Using a slotted spoon, transfer the beef in a bowl.
5. Take off the liquid from the skillet.
6. In a bowl, put together broth, ginger, flax seeds, red pepper flakes, and black pepper then mix.
7. In the same skillet, warm remaining oil on medium heat.
8. Put the carrot, broccoli, and ginger mixture then cook for at least 3-4 minutes or till desired doneness.
9. Mix in beef and scallion then cook for around 3-4 minutes.

Nutrition:

Calories: 412

Fat: 13g

Carbohydrates: 28g

Fiber: 9g

Protein: 35g

156. Beef with Mushroom & Broccoli

Preparation Time: 15 minutes

Cooking Time: 12 minutes

Servings: 4

Ingredients:

- For Beef Marinade:
- 1 garlic clove, minced
- 1 (2-inch piece fresh ginger, minced
- Salt, to taste
- Freshly ground black pepper, to taste
- 3 tbsp. white wine vinegar
- ¾ cup beef broth
- 1 lb. flank steak, trimmed and sliced into thin strips
- For Vegetables:
- 2 tbsp. coconut oil, divided
- 2 minced garlic cloves
- 3 cups broccoli rabe, chopped
- 4 oz. shiitake mushrooms halved
- 8 oz. cremini mushrooms, sliced

Directions:

1. For marinade in a bowl, put together all ingredients except beef then mix.
2. Add beef and coat with marinade.
3. Bring in the fridge to marinate for at least 15 minutes.
4. In the skillet, warm oil on medium-high heat.
5. Take off beef from the bowl, reserving the marinade.
6. Put beef and garlic and cook for about 3-4 minutes or till browned.
7. Using a slotted spoon, transfer the beef in a bowl.
8. In the same skillet, put the reserved marinade, broccoli, and mushrooms and cook for at least 3-4 minutes.
9. Stir in beef and cook for at least 3-4 minutes.

Nutrition:

Calories: 417

Fat: 10g

Carbohydrates: 23g

Fiber: 11g

Protein: 33g

157.   Citrus Beef with Bok Choy

Preparation Time: 15 minutes

Cooking Time: 11 minutes

Servings: 4

Ingredients:

- For Marinade:
- 2 minced garlic cloves
- 1 (1-inch piece fresh ginger, grated
- 1/3 cup fresh orange juice
- ½ cup coconut aminos
- 2 tsp. fish sauce
- 2 tsp. Sriracha
- 1¼ lb. sirloin steak, sliced thinly

For Veggies:

- 2 tbsp. coconut oil, divided
- 3-4 wide strips of fresh orange zest
- 1 jalapeño pepper, sliced thinly
- ½ pound string beans stemmed and halved crosswise
- 1 tbsp. arrowroot powder
- ½ pound Bok choy, chopped
- 2 tsp. sesame seeds

Directions:

1. For marinade in a big bowl, put together garlic, ginger, orange juice, coconut aminos, fish sauce, and Sriracha then mix.
2. Put the beef and coat with marinade.
3. Place in the fridge to marinate for around a couple of hours.
4. In a skillet, warm oil on medium-high heat.
5. Add orange zest and sauté approximately 2 minutes.
6. Take off the beef from a bowl, reserving the marinade.
7. In the skillet, add beef and increase the heat to high.
8. Stir fry for at least 2-3 minutes or till browned.
9. With a slotted spoon, transfer the beef and orange strips right into a bowl.
10. With a paper towel, wipe out the skillet.
11. In a similar skillet, heat remaining oil on medium-high heat.
12. Add jalapeño pepper and string beans and stir fry for about 3-4 minutes.
13. Meanwhile, add arrowroot powder in reserved marinade and stir to mix.
14. In the skillet, add marinade mixture, beef, and Bok choy and cook for about 1-2 minutes.
15. Serve hot with garnishing of sesame seeds.

Nutrition:

Calories: 398

Fat: 11g

Carbohydrates: 20g

Fiber: 6g

Protein: 34g

158.   Beef with Zucchini Noodles

Preparation Time: 15 minutes

Cooking Time: 9 minutes

Servings: 4

Ingredients:

- 1 teaspoon fresh ginger, grated
- 2 medium garlic cloves, minced
- ¼ cup coconut aminos
- 2 tablespoons fresh lime juice
- 1½ pound NY strip steak, trimmed and sliced thinly
- 2 medium zucchinis, spiralized with Blade C
- Salt, to taste
- 3 tablespoons essential olive oil
- 2 medium scallions, sliced
- 1 teaspoon red pepper flakes, crushed
- 2 tablespoons fresh cilantro, chopped

Directions:

1. In a big bowl, mix together ginger, garlic, coconut aminos, and lime juice.
2. Add beef and coat with marinade generously.
3. Refrigerate to marinate for approximately 10 minutes.
4. Place zucchini noodles over a large paper towel and sprinkle with salt.
5. Keep aside for around 10 minutes.
6. In a big skillet, heat oil on medium-high heat.
7. Add scallion and red pepper flakes and sauté for about 1 minute.
8. Add beef with marinade and stir fry for around 3-4 minutes or till browned.
9. Add zucchini and cook for approximately 3-4 minutes.
10. Serve hot with all the topping of cilantro.

Nutrition:

Calories: 434

 Fat: 17g

Carbohydrates: 23g

 Fiber: 12g

Protein: 29g

159.   Beef with Asparagus & Bell Pepper

Preparation Time: 15 minutes

Cooking Time: 13 minutes

Servings: 4-5

Ingredients:

- 4 garlic cloves, minced
- 3 tablespoons coconut aminos
- 1/8 teaspoon red pepper flakes, crushed
- 1/8 teaspoon ground ginger
- Freshly ground black pepper, to taste
- 1 bunch asparagus, trimmed and halved
- 2 tablespoons olive oil, divided
- 1-pound flank steak, trimmed and sliced thinly
- 1 red bell pepper, seeded and sliced
- 3 tablespoons water
- 2 teaspoons arrowroot powder

Directions:

1. In a bowl, mix together garlic, coconut aminos, red pepper flakes, crushed, ground ginger, and black pepper. Keep aside.
2. In a pan of boiling water, cook asparagus for about 2 minutes.
3. Drain and rinse under cold water.
4. In a substantial skillet, heat 1 tablespoon of oil on medium-high heat.
5. Add beef and stir fry for around 3-4 minutes.
6. With a slotted spoon, transfer the beef in a bowl.
7. In a similar skillet, heat remaining oil on medium heat.
8. Add asparagus and bell pepper and stir fry for approximately 2-3 minutes.
9. Meanwhile, in the bowl, mix together water and arrowroot powder.
10. Stir in beef, garlic mixture, and arrowroot mixture, and cook for around 3-4 minutes or till desired thickness.

Nutrition:

Calories: 399

Fat: 17g

Carbohydrates: 27g

Fiber: 8g

Protein: 35g

160. Spiced Ground Beef

Preparation Time: 10 minutes
Cooking Time: 22 minutes
Servings: 5
Ingredients:

- 2 tablespoons coconut oil
- 2 whole cloves
- 2 whole cardamoms
- 1 (2-inch piece cinnamon stick
- 2 bay leaves
- 1 teaspoon cumin seeds
- 2 onions, chopped
- Salt, to taste
- ½ tablespoon garlic paste
- ½ tablespoon fresh ginger paste
- 1-pound lean ground beef
- 1½ teaspoons fennel seeds powder
- 1 teaspoon ground cumin
- 1½ teaspoons red chili powder
- 1/8 teaspoon ground turmeric
- Freshly ground black pepper, to taste
- 1 cup coconut milk
- ¼ cup water
- ¼ cup fresh cilantro, chopped

Directions:

1. In a sizable pan, heat oil on medium heat.
2. Add cloves, cardamoms, cinnamon stick, bay leaves, and cumin seeds and sauté for about 20-a few seconds.
3. Add onion and 2 pinches of salt and sauté for about 3-4 minutes.
4. Add garlic-ginger paste and sauté for about 2 minutes.
5. Add beef and cook for about 4-5 minutes, entering pieces using the spoon.
6. Cover and cook approximately 5 minutes.
7. Stir in spices and cook, stirring for approximately 2-2½ minutes.
8. Stir in coconut milk and water and cook for about 7-8 minutes.
9. Season with salt and take away from heat.
10. Serve hot using the garnishing of cilantro.

Nutrition:
Calories: 444
Fat: 15g
Carbohydrates: 29g
Fiber: 11g
Protein: 39g

161.   Ground Beef with Cabbage

Preparation Time: 10 minutes

Cooking Time: 15 minutes

Servings: 6

Ingredients:

- 1 tbsp. olive oil
- 1 onion, sliced thinly
- 2 teaspoons fresh ginger, minced
- 4 garlic cloves, minced
- 1-pound lean ground beef
- 1½ tablespoons fish sauce
- 2 tablespoons fresh lime juice
- 1 small head purple cabbage, shredded
- 2 tablespoons peanut butter
- ½ cup fresh cilantro, chopped

Directions:

1. In a huge skillet, warm oil on medium heat.
2. Add onion, ginger, and garlic and sauté for about 4-5 minutes.
3. Add beef and cook for approximately 7-8 minutes, getting into pieces using the spoon.
4. Drain off the extra liquid in the skillet.
5. Stir in fish sauce and lime juice and cook for approximately 1 minute.
6. Add cabbage and cook approximately 4-5 minutes or till desired doneness.
7. Stir in peanut butter and cilantro and cook for about 1 minute.
8. Serve hot.

Nutrition:

Calories: 402

Fat: 13g

Carbohydrates: 21g

Fiber: 10g

Protein: 33g

162.   Ground Beef with Veggies

Preparation Time: 15 minutes

Cooking Time: 20 minutes

Servings: 2-4

Ingredients:

- 1-2 tablespoons coconut oil
- 1 red onion, sliced
- 2 red jalapeño peppers, seeded and sliced
- 2 minced garlic cloves
- 1-pound lean ground beef
- 1 small head broccoli, chopped
- ½ of head cauliflower, chopped
- 3 carrots, peeled and sliced
- 3 celery ribs, sliced
- Chopped fresh thyme, to taste
- Dried sage, to taste
- Ground turmeric, to taste
- Salt, to taste
- Freshly ground black pepper, to taste

Directions:

1. In a huge skillet, melt coconut oil on medium heat.
2. Add onion, jalapeño peppers and garlic and sauté for about 5 minutes.
3. Add beef and cook for around 4-5 minutes, entering pieces using the spoon.
4. Add remaining ingredients and cook, occasionally stirring for about 8-10 min.
5. Serve hot.

Nutrition:

Calories: 453

Fat: 17g

Carbohydrates: 26g

Fiber: 8g,

Protein: 35g

163.   Ground Beef with Cashews & Veggies

Preparation Time: 15 minutes

Cooking Time: 15 minutes

Servings: 4

Ingredients:

- 1½ pound lean ground beef
- 1 tablespoon garlic, minced
- 2 tablespoons fresh ginger, minced
- ¼ cup coconut aminos
- Salt, to taste
- Freshly ground black pepper, to taste
- 1 medium onion, sliced
- 1 can water chestnuts, drained and sliced
- 1 large green bell pepper, sliced
- ½ cup raw cashews, toasted

Directions:

1. Heat a nonstick skillet on medium-high heat.
2. Add beef and cook for about 6-8 minutes, breaking into pieces with all the spoon.
3. Add garlic, ginger, coconut aminos, salt, and black pepper and cook approximately 2 minutes.
4. Put the vegetables and cook approximately 5 minutes or till desired doneness.
5. Stir in cashews and immediately remove from heat.
6. Serve hot.

Nutrition:

Calories: 452

Fat: 20g

Carbohydrates: 26g

Fiber: 9g

Protein: 36g

164.   Ground Beef with Greens & Tomatoes

Preparation Time: 15 minutes

Cooking Time: 15 minutes

Servings: 4

Ingredients:

- 1 tbsp. organic olive oil
- ½ of white onion, chopped
- 2 garlic cloves, chopped finely
- 1 jalapeño pepper, chopped finely
- 1-pound lean ground beef
- 1 teaspoon ground coriander
- 1 teaspoon ground cumin
- ½ teaspoon ground turmeric
- ½ teaspoon ground ginger
- ½ teaspoon ground cinnamon
- ½ teaspoon ground fennel seeds
- Salt, to taste
- Freshly ground black pepper, to taste
- 8 fresh cherry tomatoes, quartered
- 8 collard greens leaves, stemmed and chopped
- 1 teaspoon fresh lemon juice

Directions:

1. In a huge skillet, warm oil on medium heat.
2. Put onion and sauté for approximately 4 minutes.
3. Add garlic and jalapeño pepper and sauté for approximately 1 minute.
4. Add beef and spices and cook approximately 6 minutes breaking into pieces while using spoon.
5. Stir in tomatoes and greens and cook, stirring gently for about 4 minutes.
6. Stir in lemon juice and take away from heat.

Nutrition:

Calories: 432

Fat: 16g

Carbohydrates: 27g

Fiber: 12g

Protein: 39g

165.   Beef & Veggies Chili

Preparation Time: 15 minutes

Cooking Time: 1 hour

Servings: 6-8

Ingredients:

- 2 pounds lean ground beef
- ½ head cauliflower, chopped into large pieces
- 1 onion, chopped
- 6 garlic cloves, minced
- 2 cups pumpkin puree
- 1 teaspoon dried oregano, crushed
- 1 teaspoon dried thyme, crushed
- 1 teaspoon ground cumin
- 1 teaspoon ground turmeric
- 1-2 teaspoons chili powder
- 1 teaspoon paprika
- 1 teaspoon cayenne pepper
- ¼ teaspoon red pepper flakes, crushed
- Salt, to taste
- Freshly ground black pepper, to taste
- 1 (26 oz.) can tomatoes, drained
- ½ cup water
- 1 cup beef broth

Directions:

1. Heat a substantial pan on medium-high heat.
2. Add beef and stir fry for around 5 minutes.
3. Add cauliflower, onion, and garlic and stir fry for approximately 5 minutes.
4. Add spices and herbs and stir to mix well.
5. Stir in remaining ingredients and provide to a boil.
6. Reduce heat to low and simmer, covered approximately 30-45 minutes.
7. Serve hot.

Nutrition:

Calories: 453

Fat: 10g

Carbohydrates: 20g

Fiber: 8g

Protein: 33g

166.   Ground Beef & Veggies Curry

Preparation Time: 15 minutes

Cooking Time: 36 minutes

Servings: 6-8

Ingredients:

- 2-3 tablespoons coconut oil
- 1 cup onion, chopped
- 1 garlic clove, minced
- 1-pound lean ground beef
- 1½ tablespoons curry powder
- 1/8 teaspoon ground ginger
- 1/8 teaspoon ground cinnamon
- 1/8 teaspoon ground turmeric
- Salt, to taste
- 2½-3 cups tomatoes, chopped finely
- 2½-3 cups fresh peas shelled
- 2 sweet potatoes, peeled and chopped

Directions:

1. In a sizable pan, melt coconut oil on medium heat.
2. Add onion and garlic and sauté for around 4-5 minutes.
3. Add beef and cook for about 4-5 minutes.
4. Add curry powder and spices and cook for about 1 minute.
5. Stir in tomatoes, peas, and sweet potato and bring to your gentle simmer.
6. Simmer covered approximately 25 minutes.

Nutrition:

Calorie: 432

Fat: 16g

Carbohydrates: 21g

Fiber: 11g

Protein: 36g

167.   Spicy & Creamy Ground Beef Curry

Preparation Time: 15 minutes

Cooking Time: 32 minutes

Servings: 4

Ingredients:

- 1-2 tablespoons coconut oil
- 1 teaspoon black mustard seeds
- 2 sprigs curry leaves
- 1 Serrano pepper, minced
- 1 large red onion, chopped finely
- 1 (1-inch) fresh ginger, minced
- 4 garlic cloves, minced
- 1 teaspoon ground coriander
- 1 teaspoon ground cumin
- ½ teaspoon ground turmeric
- ¼ teaspoon red chili powder
- Salt, to taste
- 1-pound lean ground beef
- 1 potato, peeled and chopped
- 3 medium carrots, peeled and chopped
- ¼ cup water
- 1 (14 oz.) can coconut milk
- Salt, to taste
- Freshly ground black pepper, to taste
- Chopped fresh cilantro, for garnishing

Directions:

1. In a big pan, melt coconut oil on medium heat.
2. Add mustard seeds and sauté for about thirty seconds.
3. Add curry leaves and Serrano pepper and sauté approximately half a minute.
4. Add onion, ginger, and garlic and sauté for about 4-5 minutes.
5. Add spices and cook for about 1 minute.
6. Add beef and cook for about 4-5 minutes.
7. Stir in potato, carrot, and water and provide with a gentle simmer.
8. Simmer, covered for around 5 minutes.
9. Stir in coconut milk and simmer for around fifteen minutes.
10. Stir in salt and black pepper and remove from heat.
11. Serve hot while using garnishing of cilantro.

Nutrition:

Calories: 432

Fat: 14g

Carbohydrates: 22g

Fiber: 8g

Protein: 39g

CHAPTER 19:

Poultry Recipes

168. Garlicky Meatballs

Preparation Time: 10 minutes
Cooking Time: 10 minutes
Servings: 2
Ingredients:

- ½ lb. boneless chicken thighs
- 1 tsp. minced garlic
- 1 ¼ cup roasted pecans
- ½ cup mushrooms
- 1 tsp. extra virgin olive oil

Directions:

1. Preheat your fryer to 375°F. Cube the chicken thighs.
2. Place them in the food processor along with the garlic, pecans, and other seasonings as desired. Pulse until a smooth consistency is achieved. Chop the mushrooms finely. Add to the chicken mixture and combine.
3. Using your hands, shape the mixture into balls and brush them with olive oil.
4. Put the balls into the fryer and cook for eighteen minutes. Serve hot.

Nutrition:

Calories: 167 Fat: 20 g Carbs: 12 g Protein: 42 g

169. Cilantro Drumsticks

Preparation Time: 12 minutes
Cooking Time: 18 minutes
Servings: 4
Ingredients:

- 8 chicken drumsticks
- ½ cup chimichurri sauce - ¼ cup lemon juice

Directions:

1. Coat the chicken drumsticks with chimichurri sauce and refrigerate in an airtight container for no less than an hour, ideally overnight.
2. When it's time to cook, pre-heat your fryer to 400°F.
3. Remove the chicken from refrigerator and allow return to room temperature for roughly twenty minutes. Cook for eighteen minutes in the fryer. Drizzle with lemon juice to taste and enjoy.

Nutrition:

Calories: 483 Fat: 29 g Carbs: 16 g Protein: 36 g

170.   Crispy Chicken

Preparation Time: 5 minutes

Cooking Time: 10 minutes

Servings: 2

Ingredients:

- 1 lb. chicken skin
- 1 tsp. butter
- ½ tsp. chili flakes
- 1 tsp. dill

Directions:

1. Pre-heat the fryer at 360°F.
2. Cut the chicken skin into slices.
3. Heat the butter until melted and pour it over the chicken skin. Toss with chili flakes, dill, and any additional seasonings to taste, making sure to coat well.
4. Cook the skins in the fryer for three minutes. Turn them over and cook on the other side for another three minutes.
5. Serve immediately or save them for later – they can be eaten hot or at room temperature.

Nutrition:

Calories: 254 Fat: 29 g Carbs: 112 g Protein: 22 g

171.   Southern Fried Chicken

Preparation Time: 5 minutes

Cooking Time: 26 minutes

Servings: 2

Ingredients:

- 2 x 6-oz. boneless skinless chicken breasts
- 2 tbsp. hot sauce
- ½ tsp. onion powder
- 1 tbsp. chili powder
- 2 oz. pork rinds, finely ground

Directions:

1. Cut the chicken breasts in half lengthwise and rub in the hot sauce. Combine the onion powder with the chili powder, then rub into the chicken. Leave to marinate for at least a half hour.
2. Use the ground pork rinds to coat the chicken breasts in the ground pork rinds, covering them thoroughly. Place the chicken in your fryer.
3. Set the fryer at 350°F and cook the chicken for 13 minutes. Flip the chicken and cook the other side for another 13 minutes or until golden.
4. Test the chicken with a meat thermometer. When fully cooked, it should reach 165°F. Serve hot, with the sides of your choice.

Nutrition:

Calories: 408 Fat: 19 g Carbs: 10 g Protein: 35 g

172. Jalapeno Chicken Breasts

Preparation Time: 5 minutes

Cooking Time: 20 minutes

Servings: 2

Ingredients:

- 2 oz. full-fat cream cheese, softened
- 4 slices sugar-free bacon, cooked and crumbled
- ¼ cup pickled jalapenos, sliced
- ½ cup sharp cheddar cheese, shredded and divided
- 2 x 6-oz. boneless skinless chicken breasts

Directions:

1. In a bowl, mix the cream cheese, bacon, jalapeno slices, and half of the cheddar cheese until well-combined.
2. Cut parallel slits in the chicken breasts of about ¾ the length – make sure not to cut all the way down. You should be able to make between six and eight slices, depending on the size of the chicken breast. Insert evenly sized dollops of the cheese mixture into the slits of the chicken breasts. Top the chicken with sprinkles of the rest of the cheddar cheese. Place the chicken in the basket of your air fryer. Set the fryer to 350°F and cook the chicken breasts for twenty minutes.
3. Test with a meat thermometer. The chicken should be at 165°F when fully cooked. Serve hot and enjoy!

Nutrition:

Calories: 276 Fat: 15 g Carbs: 11 g Protein: 24 g

173. Fajita Style Chicken Breast

Preparation Time: 10 minutes

Cooking Time: 25 minutes

Servings: 2

Ingredients:

- 2 x 6-oz. boneless skinless chicken breasts
- 1 green bell pepper, sliced
- ¼ medium white onion, sliced
- 1 tbsp. coconut oil, melted - 3 tsp. taco seasoning mix

Directions:

1. Cut each chicken breast in half and place each one between two sheets of cooking parchment. Using a mallet, pound the chicken to flatten to a quarter-inch thick. Place the chicken on a flat surface, with the short end facing you. Place four slices of pepper and three slices of onion at the end of each piece of chicken. Roll up the chicken tightly, making sure not to let any veggies fall out. Secure with some toothpicks or with butcher's string.
2. Coat the chicken with coconut oil and then with taco seasoning. Place into your air fryer.
3. Turn the fryer to 350°F and cook the chicken for twenty-five minutes. Serve the rolls immediately with your favorite dips and sides.

Nutrition:

Calories: 401 Fat: 20g Carbs: 17 g Protein: 19 g

174.   Lemon Pepper Chicken Legs

Preparation Time: 5 minutes

Cooking Time: 25 minutes

Servings: 4

Ingredients:

- ½ tsp. garlic powder
- 2 tsp. baking powder
- 8 chicken legs
- 4 tbsp. salted butter, melted
- 1 tbsp. lemon pepper seasoning

Directions:

1. In a small bowl combine the garlic powder and baking powder, then use this mixture to coat the chicken legs. Lay the chicken in the basket of your fryer.
2. Cook the chicken legs at 375°F for twenty-five minutes. Halfway through, turn them over and allow to cook on the other side.
3. When the chicken has turned golden brown, test with a thermometer to ensure it has reached an ideal temperature of 165°F. Remove from the fryer.
4. Mix together the melted butter and lemon pepper seasoning and toss with the chicken legs until the chicken is coated all over. Serve hot.

Nutrition:

Calories: 132 Fat: 16 g Carbs: 20 g Protein: 48 g

175.   Greek Chicken Meatballs

Preparation Time: 3 minutes

Cooking Time: 12 minutes

Servings: 1

Ingredients:

- ½ oz. finely ground pork rinds
- 1 lb. ground chicken
- 1 tsp. Greek seasoning
- 1/3 cup feta, crumbled
- 1/3 cup frozen spinach, drained and thawed

Directions:

1. Place all the ingredients in a large bowl and combine using your hands. Take equal-sized portions of this mixture and roll each into a 2-inch ball. Place the balls in your fryer.
2. Cook the meatballs at 350°F for twelve minutes, in several batches if necessary.
3. Once they are golden, ensure they have reached an ideal temperature of 165°F and remove from the fryer.
4. Keep each batch warm while you move on to the next one. Serve with Tzatziki if desired.

Nutrition:

Calories: 140 Fat: 43g Carbs: 25 g Protein: 12 g

176. Crusted Chicken

Preparation Time: 5 minutes

Cooking Time: 25 minutes

Servings: 2

Ingredients:

- ¼ cup slivered s
- 2x 6-oz. boneless skinless chicken breasts
- 2 tbsp. full-fat mayonnaise
- 1 tbsp. Dijon mustard

Directions:

1. Pulse the s in a food processor until they are finely chopped. Spread the s on a plate and set aside.
2. Cut each chicken breast in half lengthwise.
3. Mix the mayonnaise and mustard together and then spread evenly on top of the chicken slices. Place the chicken into the plate of chopped s to coat completely, laying each coated slice into the basket of your fryer.
4. Cook for 25 minutes at 350°F until golden. Test the temperature, making sure the chicken has reached 165°F. Serve hot.

Nutrition:

Calories: 204 Fat: 30 g Carbs: 14 g Protein: 23 g

177. Buffalo Chicken Tenders

Preparation Time: 12 minutes

Cooking Time: 8 minutes

Servings: 4

Ingredients:

- 1 egg
- 1 cup mozzarella cheese, shredded
- ¼ cup buffalo sauce
- 1 cup cooked chicken, shredded
- ¼ cup feta cheese

Directions:

1. Combine all ingredients (except for the feta). Line the basket of your fryer with a suitably sized piece of parchment paper. Lay the mixture into the fryer and press it into a circle about half an inch thick. Crumble the feta cheese over it.
2. Cook for eight minutes at 400°F. Turn the fryer off and allow the chicken to rest inside before removing with care.
3. Cut the mixture into slices and serve hot.

Nutrition:

Calories: 240 Fat: 10g Carbs: 20 g Protein: 20 g

178.   Buffalo Chicken Strips

Preparation Time: 5 minutes

Cooking Time: 25 minutes

Servings: 1

Ingredients:

- ¼ cup hot sauce
- 1 lb. boneless skinless chicken tenders
- 1 tsp. garlic powder
- 1 ½ oz. pork rinds, finely ground
- 1 tsp chili powder

Directions:

1. Toss the hot sauce and chicken tenders together in a bowl, ensuring the chicken is completely coated.
2. In another bowl, combine the garlic powder, ground pork rinds, and chili powder. Use this mixture to coat the tenders, covering them well. Place the chicken into your fryer, taking care not to layer pieces on top of one another.
3. Cook the chicken at 375°F for twenty minutes until cooked all the way through and golden. Serve warm with your favorite dips and sides.

Nutrition:

Calories: 143 Fat: 29 g Carbs: 15 g Protein: 30 g

179.   Chicken & Pepperoni Pizza

Preparation Time: 5 minutes

Cooking Time: 15 minutes

Servings: 6

Ingredients:

- 2 cups cooked chicken, cubed
- 20 slices pepperoni
- 1 cup sugar-free pizza sauce
- 1 cup mozzarella cheese, shredded
- ¼ cup parmesan cheese, grated

Directions:

1. Place the chicken into the base of a four-cup baking dish and add the pepperoni and pizza sauce on top. Mix well so as to completely coat the meat with the sauce.
2. Add the parmesan and mozzarella on top of the chicken, then place the baking dish into your fryer.
3. Cook for 15 minutes at 375°F.
4. When everything is bubbling and melted, remove from the fryer. Serve hot.

Nutrition:

Calories: 239 Fat: 12 g

Carbs: 8 g Protein: 11 g

180.   Italian Chicken Thighs

Preparation Time: 10 minutes
Cooking Time: 20 minutes
Servings: 4

Ingredients:

- 4 skin-on bone-in chicken thighs
- 2 tbsp. unsalted butter, melted
- 3 tsp. Italian herbs
- ½ tsp. garlic powder
- ¼ tsp. onion powder

Directions:

1. Using a brush, coat the chicken thighs with the melted butter. Combine the herbs with the garlic powder and onion powder, then massage into the chicken thighs. Place the thighs in the fryer.
2. Cook at 380°F for 20 minutes, turning the chicken halfway through to cook on the other side.
3. When the thighs have achieved a golden color, test the temperature with a meat thermometer. Once they have reached 165°F, remove from the fryer and serve.

Nutrition:

Calories: 265

Fat: 21 g

Carbs: 22 g

Protein: 32 g

CHAPTER 20:

Poultry

181.   Egg White Vegetable Scramble

Preparation Time: 5 minutes

Cooking Time: 10 minutes

Servings: 5

Ingredients:

- Olive or cooking oil
- 6 large eggs
- 1/2 cup of chopped fresh mushrooms
- 1/2 cup of chopped fresh broccoli florets
- 1/2 cup diced orange pepper and red pepper
- Fresh spinach/vegetables
- 1% or 2% of milk
- Grated cheese (optional)
- 1/5 teaspoon of grounded black pepper
- A pinch of salt
- Onions
- Cooking oil, either butter flavored or olive oil
- Tomatoes

Directions:

1. Over medium heat, heat your oil in a frying pan
2. Add your fresh mushrooms, onions, broccoli florets, pepper and salts, don't stop stirring until your onions are transparent
3. Beat 6 large eggs and milk in a mixing bowl and mix well
4. Add your egg mixture to your vegetables or spinach
5. Stir in your tomatoes
6. Mix in the cheese when you notice the eggs are almost done.
7. Then serve immediately

Nutrition:

Fat: 12.4 g Cholesterol: 15 mg Sodium: 371.6 mg

Potassium: 138.6 mg Carbohydrate: 6 g Protein: 20.8 g

182. Egg and Potato Strata

Preparation Time: 20 minutes

Cooking Time: 6 to 8 hours

Servings: 8

Ingredients:

- 8 Yukon Gold potatoes, peeled and diced
- 1 onion, minced
- 2 red bell peppers, stemmed, seeded, and minced
- 3 Roma tomatoes, seeded and chopped
- 3 garlic cloves, minced
- 11/2 cups shredded Swiss cheese
- 8 eggs
- 2 egg whites
- 1 teaspoon dried marjoram leaves
- 1 cup 2% milk

Directions:

1. In a 6-quart slow cooker, layer the diced potatoes, onion, bell peppers, tomatoes, garlic, and cheese.
2. In a medium bowl, mix the eggs, egg whites, marjoram, and milk well with a wire whisk. Pour this mixture into the slow cooker.
3. Cover and cook on low for 6 to 8 hours, do it until a food thermometer registers 165°F and the potatoes are tender.
4. Scoop out of the slow cooker to serve.

Nutrition:

Calories: 305 Cal

Carbohydrates: 33 g

Sugar: 5 g

Fiber: 3 g

Fat: 12 g

Saturated Fat: 6 g

Protein: 17 g

Sodium: 136 mg

183.   Scrambled Eggs with Goat Cheese and Roasted Peppers

Preparation Time: 5 minutes

Cooking Time: 10 minutes

Servings: 4

Ingredients:

- 11/2 teaspoons extra-virgin olive oil
- 1 cup chopped bell peppers, any color (about 1 medium pepper)
- 2 garlic cloves, minced (about 1 teaspoon)
- 6 large eggs
- 1/4 teaspoon kosher or sea salt
- 2 tablespoons water
- 1/2 cup crumbled goat cheese (about 2 ounces)
- 2 tablespoons loosely packed chopped fresh mint

Directions:

- In a large skillet over medium-high heat, heat the oil. Add the peppers and cook for 5 minutes, stirring occasionally.
- Add the garlic and cook for 1 minute.
- While the peppers are cooking, they whisk together the eggs, salt, and water in a medium bowl.
- Turn the heat down to medium-low.
- Pour the egg mixture over the peppers.
- Let the eggs cook undisturbed for 1 to 2 minutes, until they begin to set on the bottom.
- Sprinkle with the goat cheese.
- Cook the eggs for about 1 to 2 more minutes, stirring slowly, until the eggs are soft-set and custardy.
- Top with the fresh mint and serve.

Nutrition:

Calories: 201 Cal

Fat: 15 g

Cholesterol: 294 mg

Sodium: 176 mg

Carbohydrates: 5 g

Fiber: 2 g

Protein: 15 g

184. Marinara Eggs with Parsley

Preparation Time: 5 minutes

Cooking Time: 15 minutes

Servings: 6

Ingredients:

- 1 tablespoon extra-virgin olive oil
- 1 cup chopped onion (about 1/2 medium onion)
- 2 garlic cloves, minced (about 1 teaspoon)
- 2 (14.5-ounce) cans Italian diced tomatoes, undrained, no salt added
- 6 large eggs
- 1/2 cup chopped fresh flat-leaf (Italian) parsley
- Crusty Italian bread and grated Parmesan or Romano cheese, for serving (optional)

Directions:

1. In a large skillet over medium-high heat, heat the oil.
2. Add the onion and cook for 5 minutes, stirring occasionally.
3. Add the garlic and cook for 1 minute.
4. Pour the tomatoes with their juices over the onion mixture and cook until bubbling, 2 to 3 minutes.
5. While waiting for the tomato mixture to bubble, crack one egg into a small custard cup or coffee mug.
6. When the tomato mixture bubbles, lower the heat to medium.
7. Then use a large spoon to make six indentations in the tomato mixture.
8. Gently pour the first cracked egg into one indentation and repeat, cracking the remaining eggs, one at a time, into the custard cup and pouring one into each indentation.
9. Cover the skillet and cook for 6 to 7 minutes, or until the eggs are done to your liking (about 6 minutes for soft-cooked, 7 minutes for harder cooked).
10. Top with the parsley, and serve with the bread and grated cheese, if desired.

Nutrition:

Calories: 122 Cal

Fat: 7 g

Cholesterol: 186 mg

Sodium: 207 mg

Carbohydrates: 7 g

Fiber: 1 g

Protein: 7 g

185.   Quinoa-Kale Egg Casserole

Preparation Time: 20 minutes

Cooking Time: 6 to 8 hours

Servings: 8

Ingredients:

- 11/2 cups roasted vegetable broth
- 11 eggs
- 11/2 cups quinoa, rinsed and drained
- 3 cups chopped kale
- 1 leek, chopped
- 1 red bell pepper, stemmed, seeded, and chopped
- 3 garlic cloves, minced
- 11/2 cups shredded Havarti cheese

Directions:

1. Grease a 6-quart slow cooker with vegetable oil and set aside.
2. In a large bowl, mix the milk, vegetable broth, and eggs and beat well with a wire whisk.
3. Stir in the quinoa, kale, leek, bell pepper, garlic, and cheese. Pour this mixture into the prepared slow cooker.
4. Cover and cook on low for 6 to 8 hours, or until a food thermometer registers 165°F and the mixture is set.

Nutrition:

Calories: 483 Cal

Carbohydrates: 32 g

Sugar: 8 g

Fiber: 3 g

Fat: 27 g

Saturated Fat: 14 g

Protein: 25 g

Sodium: 462 mg

186. Chicken and Pasta Casserole

Preparation Time: 15 minutes

Cooking Time: 20 minutes

Servings: 6

Ingredients:

- 8 ounces dry fusilli pasta
- 1 1/2 ounces olive oil
- 6 chicken tenderloins, cut in bite-sized chunks
- 1 tablespoon dried minced onion
- A pinch of salt and pepper
- A bit of garlic powder
- ½ ounce basil, dried
- ½ ounce parsley, dried
- 10 3/4 ounces condensed cream of chicken soup
- 10 3/4 ounces condensed cream of mushroom soup
- 16 ounces frozen mixed vegetables
- 8 ounces bread crumbs
- 1-ounce Parmesan cheese, grated
- 1-ounce melted butter

Directions:

1. Preheat oven to 400 degrees Fahrenheit.
2. Lightly coat a baking dish with cooking spray.
3. Boil a large pot of salted water and cook fusilli noodles for 10 minutes or until tender but firm to the bite.
4. Drain water out of the pot.
5. Heat oil in a large frying pan on medium heat. Cook chicken in the oil with onion, salt, pepper, garlic powder, basil, and parsley for 20 minutes or until juices run clear.
6. Stir in pasta, soups and vegetables. Pour the mixture into the baking dish.
7. Mix bread crumbs, parmesan and butter in a small bowl and spread over the pasta.
8. Bake for 20 minutes or until browned and bubbly.

Nutrition:

Calories: 416 Cal

Carbohydrates: 33 g

Sugar: 18 g

Fiber: 15 g

187.   Egg and Wild Rice Casserole

Preparation Time: 20 minutes

Cooking Time: 5 to 7 hours

Servings: 6

Ingredients:

- 3 cups plain cooked wild rice or Herbed Wild Rice
- 2 cups sliced mushrooms
- 1 red bell pepper, stemmed, seeded, and chopped
- 1 onion, minced
- 2 garlic cloves, minced
- 11 eggs
- 1 teaspoon dried thyme leaves
- 1/4 teaspoon salt
- 11/2 cups shredded Swiss cheese

Directions:

1. In a 6-quart slow cooker, layer the wild rice, mushrooms, bell pepper, onion, and garlic.
2. In a large bowl, beat the eggs with the thyme and salt. Pour into the slow cooker. Top with the cheese.
3. Cover and cook on low for 5 to 7 hours, or until a food thermometer registers 165°F and the casserole is set.

Nutrition:

Calories: 360 Cal

Carbohydrates: 25 g

Sugar: 3 g

Fiber: 3 g

Fat: 17 g

Saturated Fat: 8 g

Protein: 24 g

Sodium: 490 mg

188.   Turkey Spinach Egg Muffins

Preparation Time: 10 minutes

Cooking Time: 30 minutes

Servings: 3

Ingredients:

- 5 egg whites
- 2 eggs
- 1/4 cup cheddar cheese, shredded
- 1/4 cup spinach, chopped
- 1/4 cup milk
- 3 lean breakfast turkey sausage
- Pepper
- Salt

Directions:

1. Preheat the oven to 350 F.
2. Grease muffin tray cups and set aside.
3. In a pan, brown the turkey sausage links over medium-high heat until the sausage is brown from all the sides.
4. Cut sausage in 1/2-inch pieces and set aside.
5. In a large bowl, whisk together eggs, egg whites, milk, pepper, and salt.
6. Stir in the spinach.
7. Pour the egg mixture into the prepared muffin tray.
8. Divide the sausage and the cheese evenly between each muffin cup.
9. Bake in preheated oven for 20 minutes or until muffins are set.
10. Serve warm and enjoy.

Nutrition:

Calories: 123 Cal

Fat: 6.8 g

Carbohydrates: 1.9 g

Sugar: 1.6 g

Protein: 13.3 g

Cholesterol: 123 mg

189.   Cheesy Egg Veggie Omelet

Preparation Time: 5 minutes

Cooking Time: 6 minutes

Servings: 2

Ingredients:

- 3 eggs
- 1/2 cup cheddar cheese, grated
- 2 garlic cloves, minced
- 1 tbsp. parsley, chopped
- Sea salt and pepper to taste
- 2 tbsp. mozzarella cheese, grated
- 1 tbsp. olive oil

Directions:

1. Whisk the eggs in a bowl. Add some salt and pepper.
2. Heat the olive oil in a pan.
3. Add the garlic and toss for 1 minute.
4. Add the egg mixture and cook for 1 minute.
5. Add the cheddar, parsley, and parmesan cheese.
6. Fold the egg in half and cook for another minute.
7. Serve hot.

Nutrition:

Protein: 21.7 g

Carbohydrates: 9.1 g

Dietary Fiber: 1.6 g

Sugars: 4.8 g

Fat: 29.8 g

190.   Egg Avocado Toast

Preparation Time: 5 minutes

Cooking Time: 5 minutes

Servings: 2

Ingredients:

- 2 almond bread slices
- 2 eggs
- 1 cup avocado puree
- Sea salt to taste
- 1 tbsp. almond butter
- Cayenne pepper to taste
- 1 tsp. chives, chopped

Directions:

1. Toast the bread slices.
2. Spread the avocado puree onto the bread slices.
3. In a pan, add the almond butter and melt over medium heat.
4. Add the eggs and whisk for 1 minute.
5. Add the salt and cayenne pepper.
6. Scramble for 1 minute and add on top of the toast.
7. Add the chives, more salt, and pepper on top.

Nutrition:

Fat: 18.2 g

Carbohydrates: 19.3 g

Fiber: 9.8 g

Protein: 14.6 g

Sugar: 2.9 g

Sodium: 252 mg

191.   Egg Mushroom Omelet

Preparation Time: 5 minutes

Cooking Time: 5 minutes

Servings: 2

Ingredients:

- 3 eggs
- 1 cup button mushroom, chopped
- 1 baby shallot, chopped
- Sea salt to taste
- Cayenne pepper to taste
- 1 tbsp. olive oil

Directions:

1. In a mixing bowl, beat the eggs with sea salt, cayenne pepper.
2. Heat the oil in a skillet over medium heat.
3. Pour in the egg mixture.
4. Cook for 1 minute and add the mushroom and shallots.
5. Cover and cook for 2 minutes. Take off the heat and serve.

Nutrition:

Fat: 75 g Protein: 18 g Sodium: 195 mg

192.   Chicken Salad with Pineapple and Pecans

Preparation Time: 10 minutes

Cooking Time: 5 minutes

Servings: 4

Ingredients:

- (6-ounce) Boneless, skinless, cooked and cubed chicken breast
- Celery
- 1/4 cup of pineapple
- 1/4 cup orange, peeled segments
- Tablespoon of pecans
- 1/4 cup seedless grapes
- Salt and black chili pepper, to taste
- Cups cut from roman lettuce

Directions:

1. Put chicken, celery, pineapple, grapes, pecans, and raisins in a medium dish.
2. Kindly blend until mixed with a spoon, then season with salt and pepper.
3. Create a bed of lettuce on a plate. Cover with mixture of chicken and serve.

Nutrition:

Calories: 386 Cal Carbohydrates: 20 g Fat: 19 g Protein: 25 g

CHAPTER 21:

Snacks

193.   Cucumber Sandwich Bites

Preparation Time: 5 minutes
Cooking Time: 0 minutes
Servings: 12
Ingredients:

- 1 cucumber, sliced
- 8 slices whole wheat bread
- 2 tablespoons cream cheese, soft
- 1 tablespoon chives, chopped
- ¼ cup avocado, peeled, pitted and mashed
- 1 teaspoon mustard
- Salt and black pepper to the taste

Directions:

1. Spread the mashed avocado on each bread slice, also spread the rest of the ingredients except the cucumber slices.
2. Divide the cucumber slices on the bread slices, cut each slice in thirds, arrange on a platter and serve as an appetizer.

Nutrition:

Calories 187;

Fat 12.4 g;

Fiber 2.1 g;

Carbs 4.5 g;

Protein 8.2 g

194.   Cucumber Rolls

Preparation Time: 5 minutes

Cooking Time: 0 minutes

Servings: 6

Ingredients:

- 1 big cucumber, sliced lengthwise
- 1 tablespoon parsley, chopped
- 8 ounces canned tuna, drained and mashed
- Salt and black pepper to the taste
- 1 teaspoon lime juice

Directions:

1. Arrange cucumber slices on a working surface, divide the rest of the ingredients, and roll.
2. Arrange all the rolls on a platter and serve as an appetizer.

Nutrition:

Calories 200

Fat 6 g

Fiber 3.4 g

Carbs 7.6 g

Protein 3.5 g

195.   Olives and Cheese Stuffed Tomatoes

Preparation Time: 10 minutes

Cooking Time: 0 minutes

Servings: 24

Ingredients:

- 24 cherry tomatoes, top cut off and insides scooped out
- 2 tablespoons olive oil
- ¼ teaspoon red pepper flakes
- ½ cup feta cheese, crumbled
- 2 tablespoons black olive paste
- ¼ cup mint, torn

Directions:

1. In a bowl, mix the olives paste with the rest of the ingredients except the cherry tomatoes and whisk well.
2. Stuff the cherry tomatoes with this mix, arrange them all on a platter and serve as an appetizer.

Nutrition:

Calories 136;

Fat 8.6 g;

Fiber 4.8 g;

Carbs 5.6 g;

Protein 5.1 g

196.   Tomato Salsa

Preparation Time: 5 minutes

Cooking Time: 0 minutes

Servings: 6

Ingredients:

- 1 garlic clove, minced
- 4 tablespoons olive oil
- 5 tomatoes, cubed
- 1 tablespoon balsamic vinegar
- ¼ cup basil, chopped
- 1 tablespoon parsley, chopped
- 1 tablespoon chives, chopped
- Salt and black pepper to the taste
- Pita chips for serving

Directions:

1. In a bowl, mix the tomatoes with the garlic and the rest of the ingredients except the pita chips, stir, divide into small cups and serve with the pita chips on the side.

Nutrition:

Calories 160; Fat 13.7 g; Fiber 5.5 g; Carbs 10.1 g; Protein 2.2

197.   Chili Mango and Watermelon Salsa

Preparation Time: 5 minutes

Cooking Time: 0 minutes

Servings: 12

Ingredients:

- 1 red tomato, chopped
- Salt and black pepper to the taste
- 1 cup watermelon, seedless, peeled and cubed
- 1 red onion, chopped
- 2 mangos, peeled and chopped
- 2 chili peppers, chopped
- ¼ cup cilantro, chopped
- 3 tablespoons lime juice
- Pita chips for serving

Directions:

1. In a bowl, mix the tomato with the watermelon, the onion and the rest of the ingredients except the pita chips and toss well.
2. Divide the mix into small cups and serve with pita chips on the side.

Nutrition:

Calories 62; Fat 4g; Fiber 1.3 g; Carbs 3.9 g; Protein 2.3 g

198.   Creamy Spinach and Shallots Dip

Preparation Time: 10 minutes

Cooking Time: 0 minutes

Servings: 4

Ingredients:

- 1 pound spinach, roughly chopped
- 2 shallots, chopped
- 2 tablespoons mint, chopped
- ¾ cup cream cheese, soft
- Salt and black pepper to the taste

Directions:

1. In a blender, combine the spinach with the shallots and the rest of the ingredients, and pulse well.
2. Divide into small bowls and serve as a party dip.

Nutrition:

Calories 204;

Fat 11.5 g;

Fiber 3.1 g;

Carbs 4.2 g;

Protein 5.9 g

199.   Feta Artichoke Dip

Preparation Time: 10 minutes

Cooking Time: 30 minutes

Servings: 8

Ingredients:

- 8 ounces artichoke hearts, drained and quartered
- ¾ cup basil, chopped
- ¾ cup green olives, pitted and chopped
- 1 cup parmesan cheese, grated
- 5 ounces feta cheese, crumbled

Directions:

1. In your food processor, mix the artichokes with the basil and the rest of the ingredients, pulse well, and transfer to a baking dish.
2. Introduce in the oven, bake at 375° F for 30 minutes and serve as a party dip.

Nutrition:

Calories 186;

Fat 12.4 g;

Fiber 0.9 g;

Carbs 2.6 g;

Protein 1.5 g

200. Avocado Dip

Preparation Time: 5 minutes

Cooking Time: 0 minutes

Servings: 8

Ingredients:

- ½ cup heavy cream
- 1 green chili pepper, chopped
- Salt and pepper to the taste
- 4 avocados, pitted, peeled and chopped
- 1 cup cilantro, chopped
- ¼ cup lime juice

Directions:

1. In a blender, combine the cream with the avocados and the rest of the ingredients and pulse well.
2. Divide the mix into bowls and serve cold as a party dip.

Nutrition:

Calories 200;

Fat 14.5 g;

Fiber 3.8 g;

Carbs 8.1 g;

Protein 7.6 g

201. Goat Cheese and Chives Spread

Preparation Time: 10 minutes

Cooking Time: 0 minute

Servings: 4

Ingredients:

- 2 ounces goat cheese, crumbled
- ¾ cup sour cream
- 2 tablespoons chives, chopped
- 1 tablespoon lemon juice
- Salt and black pepper to the taste
- 2 tablespoons extra virgin olive oil

Directions:

1. In a bowl, mix the goat cheese with the cream and the rest of the ingredients and whisk really well.
2. Keep in the fridge for 10 minutes and serve as a party spread.

Nutrition:

Calories 220;

Fat 11.5 g;

Fiber 4.8 g;

Carbs 8.9 g;

Protein 5.6 g

202. White Bean Dip

Preparation Time: 10 minutes
Cooking Time: 0 minute
Servings: 4
Ingredients:

- 15 ounces canned white beans, drained and rinsed
- 6 ounces canned artichoke hearts, drained and quartered
- 4 garlic cloves, minced
- 1 tablespoon basil, chopped
- 2 tablespoons olive oil
- Juice of ½ lemon
- Zest of ½ lemon, grated
- Salt and black pepper to the taste

Directions:

1. In your food processor, combine the beans with the artichokes and the rest of the ingredients except the oil and pulse well.
2. Add the oil gradually, pulse the mix again, divide into cups and serve as a party dip.

Nutrition:

Calories 274; Fat 11.7 g; Fiber 6.5 g; Carbs 18.5 g; Protein 16.5 g

203. Eggplant Dip

Preparation Time: 10 minutes
Cooking Time: 40 minutes
Servings: 4
Ingredients:

- 1 eggplant, poked with a fork
- 2 tablespoons tahini paste
- 2 tablespoons lemon juice
- 2 garlic cloves, minced
- 1 tablespoon olive oil
- Salt and black pepper to the taste
- 1 tablespoon parsley, chopped

Directions:

1. Put the eggplant in a roasting pan, bake at 400° F for 40 minutes, cool down, peel and transfer to your food processor.
2. Add the rest of the ingredients except the parsley, pulse well, divide into small bowls and serve as an appetizer with the parsley sprinkled on top.

Nutrition:

Calories 121; Fat 4.3 g; Fiber 1 g; Carbs 1.4 g; Protein 4.3 g

204.   Bulgur Lamb Meatballs

Preparation Time: 10 minutes

Cooking Time: 15 minute

Servings: 6

Ingredients:

- 1 and ½ cups Greek yogurt
- ½ teaspoon cumin, ground
- 1 cup cucumber, shredded
- ½ teaspoon garlic, minced
- A pinch of salt and black pepper
- 1 cup bulgur
- 2 cups water
- 1 pound lamb, ground
- ¼ cup parsley, chopped
- ¼ cup shallots, chopped
- ½ teaspoon allspice, ground
- ½ teaspoon cinnamon powder
- 1 tablespoon olive oil

Directions:

1. In a bowl, combine the bulgur with the water, cover the bowl, leave aside for 10 minutes, drain and transfer to a bowl.
2. Add the meat, the yogurt and the rest of the ingredients except the oil, stir well and shape medium meatballs out of this mix.
3. Heat up a pan with the oil over medium-high heat, add the meatballs, cook them for 7 minutes on each side, arrange them all on a platter and serve as an appetizer.

Nutrition:

Calories 300;

Fat 9.6 g;

Fiber 4.6 g;

Carbs 22.6 g;

Protein 6.6 g

205.   Cucumber Bites

Preparation Time: 10 minutes

Cooking Time: 0 minutes

Servings: 12

Ingredients:

- 1 English cucumber, sliced into 32 rounds
- 10 ounces hummus
- 16 cherry tomatoes, halved
- 1 tablespoon parsley, chopped
- 1 ounce feta cheese, crumbled

Directions:

1. Spread the hummus on each cucumber round, divide the tomato halves on each, sprinkle the cheese and parsley on to and serve as an appetizer.

Nutrition:

Calories 162;

Fat 3.4 g;

Fiber 2 g;

Carbs 6.4 g;

Protein 2.4 g

206.   Stuffed Avocado

Preparation Time: 10 minutes

Cooking Time: 0 minute

Servings: 2

Ingredients:

- 1 avocado, halved and pitted
- 10 ounces canned tuna, drained
- 2 tablespoons sun-dried tomatoes, chopped
- 1 and ½ tablespoon basil pesto
- 2 tablespoons black olives, pitted and chopped
- Salt and black pepper to the taste
- 2 teaspoons pine nuts, toasted and chopped
- 1 tablespoon basil, chopped

Directions:

1. In a bowl, combine the tuna with the sun-dried tomatoes and the rest of the ingredients except the avocado and stir.
2. Stuff the avocado halves with the tuna mix and serve as an appetizer.

Nutrition:

Calories 233; Fat 9 g; Fiber 3.5 g; Carbs 11.4 g; Protein 5.6 g

207.   Hummus with Ground Lamb

Preparation Time: 10 minutes

Cooking Time: 15 minute

Servings: 8

Ingredients:

- 10 ounces hummus
- 12 ounces lamb meat, ground
- ½ cup pomegranate seeds
- ¼ cup parsley, chopped
- 1 tablespoon olive oil
- Pita chips for serving

Directions:

1. Heat up a pan with the oil over medium-high heat, add the meat, and brown for 15 minutes stirring often.
2. Spread the hummus on a platter, spread the ground lamb all over, also spread the pomegranate seeds and the parsley and serve with pita chips as a snack.

Nutrition:

Calories 133;

Fat 9.7 g;

Fiber 1.7 g;

Carbs 6.4 g;

Protein 5

208.   Wrapped Plums

Preparation Time: 5 minutes

Cooking Time: 0 minutes

Servings: 8

Ingredients:

- 2 ounces prosciutto, cut into 16 pieces
- 4 plums, quartered
- 1 tablespoon chives, chopped
- A pinch of red pepper flakes, crushed

Directions:

3. Wrap each plum quarter in a prosciutto slice, arrange them all on a platter, sprinkle the chives and pepper flakes all over and serve.

Nutrition:

Calories 30;

Fat 1 g;

Fiber 0 g;

Carbs 4 g;

Protein 2 g

Conclusion

The fact that the Optavia program is appropriate for many, many people speaks for such a diet in its favor. It is an isolated enough problem to not be of too much concern for most. You may also not have an issue with putting Optavia in your body and keep a healthy weight even if you adjust your eating habits. This diet deserves credit for being a legitimately well-formulated reduction plan by addressing various aspects of the fad with proven research, a plan that is definitely fitted for the individual.

Anyone who's tried should understand that discovering the best diet of any kind can be somewhat of a challenge. The fact that there's seemly infinite ways to help you lose weight by strict diets, weight loss pills, programs, fads, gimmicks, and everything in between, can all-too-easily be overwhelming and choose you or more likely. With so many different diet plans like the Optavia Diet coming onto the market, there's a lot of talk about which one really works. The goal of this article is to give an honest review regarding this new diet, and determine whether it's worth your time or money.

As effective as this meal plan is, there are some risks that have also been discussed nonetheless. A far as weight reduction goes, experts agree that while Optavia can benefit its users because it's lower in calories, for the better, it's unlikely to significantly change your eating habits. You're more prone to regain the weight back once you quit your regimen. So, if, as a result of having gone through the plan, a person ends up modifying their eating patterns to eliminate certain unhealthy foods and maintains a healthy weight, it would be an independent beneficial element coming out of this diet– like the cherry on top.

The gist of the book is that to lose weight you have to be on a meal plan. You follow the menu found on the packaging and you cannot deviate from the route. This isn't meant to be a thigh-slapper for our "health-conscious" society. It's a main part of the plan, so that you can lose weight. You're meant to be on the diet for eight weeks, but there is a fourteen-day free trial period available so that you can try it out and see how it works for you.

You're instructed to cut calories, not medications. You're not going to lose thirty pounds in a week. You're not going to find it under the sofa or in the back of your closet. If you're following the chart, there won't be any leftovers.

The diet is carefully targeted at recording the calories you take in, as well as the calories you expel. There are waste-emissions from your body, gas, and other nuisances. You're not going to be able to choose which of those to lose, so the more of them you get rid of, the more weight you're going to lose.

The program is clear cut, so you know exactly what you're going to eat, and you know exactly what it's going to cost. There are no surprises, you can use your mobile phone to check your app, and you can look at the shopping list on the website.

CPSIA information can be obtained
at www.ICGtesting.com
Printed in the USA
LVHW050342180121
676772LV00011B/388

9 781801 545495